Nathaniel J. Pallone
Editor

Treating Substance Abusers in Correctional Contexts: New Understandings, New Modalities

Treating Substance Abusers in Correctional Contexts: New Understandings, New Modalities has been co-published simultaneously as *Journal of Offender Rehabilitation*, Volume 37, Numbers 3/4 2003.

Pre-publication
REVIEWS,
COMMENTARIES,
EVALUATIONS . . .

"INTRIGUING AND ILLUMINATING. . . . Includes qualitative and quantitative research on juvenile and adult-oriented programs in the United States, Britain, and Hong Kong. . . . Examines a multitude of issues relevant to substance abuse treatment in the criminal justice system. . . . Also includes several chapters examining the effectiveness of drug courts. . . . Provides some answers to the questions being asked about RSAT programs and highlights what may be the most intriguing and encouraging development in corrections in the past quarter-century. I HIGHLY RECOMMEND THIS BOOK to anyone interested in substance abuse treatment programs."

Craig Hemmens, JD, PhD
Chair and Associate Professor
Department of Criminal Justice
Administration, Boise State University

The Haworth Press, Inc.

Treating Substance Abusers in Correctional Contexts: New Understandings, New Modalities

Treating Substance Abusers in Correctional Contexts: New Understandings, New Modalities has been co-published simultaneously as *Journal of Offender Rehabilitation*, Volume 37, Numbers 3/4 2003.

The *Journal of Offender Rehabilitation* Monographic "Separates"

Below is a list of "separates," which in serials librarianship means a special issue simultaneously published as a special journal issue or double-issue *and* as a "separate" hardbound monograph. (This is a format which we also call a "DocuSerial.")

"Separates" are published because specialized libraries or professionals may wish to purchase a specific thematic issue by itself in a format which can be separately cataloged and shelved, as opposed to purchasing the journal on an on-going basis. Faculty members may also more easily consider a "separate" for classroom adoption.

"Separates" are carefully classified separately with the major book jobbers so that the journal tie-in can be noted on new book order slips to avoid duplicate purchasing.

You may wish to visit Haworth's website at . . .

http://www.HaworthPress.com

. . . to search our online catalog for complete tables of contents of these separates and related publications.

You may also call 1-800-HAWORTH (outside US/Canada: 607-722-5857), or Fax 1-800-895-0582 (outside US/Canada: 607-771-0012), or e-mail at:

docdelivery@haworthpress.com

Treating Substance Abusers in Correctional Contexts: New Understandings, New Modalities, edited by Nathaniel J. Pallone, PhD (Vol. 37, No. 3/4, 2003). *"Intriguing and illuminating. . . . Includes qualitative and quantitative research on juvenile and adult-oriented programs in the United States, Britain, and Hong Kong. . . . Examines a multitude of issues relevant to substance abuse treatment in the criminal justice system. . . . Also includes several chapters examining the effectiveness of drug courts. . . . Provides some answers to the questions being asked about RSAT programs and highlights what may be the most intriguing and encouraging development in corrections in the past quarter-century. I highly recommend this book to anyone interested in substance abuse treatment programs." (Craig Hemmens, JD, PhD, Chair and Associate Professor, Department of Criminal Justice Administration, Boise State University)*

Transcendental Meditation® in Criminal Rehabilitation and Crime Prevention, edited by Charles N. Alexander, PhD, Kenneth G. Walton, PhD, David W. Orme-Johnson, PhD, Rachel S. Goodman, PhD, and Nathaniel J. Pallone, PhD (Vol. 36, No. 1/2/3/4, 2003). *"Makes a strong case that meditation can accelerate development in adult criminal populations, leading to reduced recidivism and other favorable outcomes. . . . Contains original research and reviews of over 25 studies that demonstrate the effectiveness of TM programs in criminal rehabilitation." (Juan Pascual-Leone, MD, PhD, Professor of Psychology, York University)*

Religion, the Community, and the Rehabilitation of Criminal Offenders, edited by Thomas P. O'Connor, BCL, BTheol, MS, and Nathaniel J. Pallone, PhD (Vol. 35, No. 3/4, 2002). *Examines the relationship between faith-based programs, religion, and offender rehabilitation.*

Drug Courts in Operation: Current Research, edited by James J. Hennessy, PhD, and Nathaniel J. Pallone, PhD (Vol. 33, No. 4, 2001). *"As one of the founders of the drug court movement, I can testify that Dr. Hennessy's book represents the highest level of sophistication in this field." (Michael O. Smith, MD, Director, Lincoln Recovery Center, Bronx, New York; Assistant Clinical Professor of Psychiatry, Cornell University Medical School)*

Family Empowerment as an Intervention Strategy in Juvenile Delinquency, edited by Richard Dembo, PhD, and Nathaniel J. Pallone, PhD (Vol. 33, No. 1, 2001). *"A hands-on book. . . . Provides detailed guidelines for counselors regarding implementation of the FEI curriculum . . . accurately describes the scope of counselor responsibilities and the nature of treatment interventions. Unique in its coverage of counselor competencies and training/supervision needs. Innovative and based on solid empirical evidence." (Roger H. Peters, PhD, Professor, University of South Florida, Tampa)*

Race, Ethnicity, Sexual Orientation, Violent Crime: The Realities and the Myths, edited by Nathaniel J. Pallone, PhD (Vol. 30, No. 1/2, 1999). *"A fascinating book which illuminates the complexity of race as it applies to the criminal justice system and the myths and political correctness that have shrouded the real truth. . . . I highly recommend this book for those who study causes of crime in minority populations." (Joseph R. Carlson, PhD, Associate Professor, University of Nebraska at Kearney)*

Sex Offender Treatment: Biological Dysfunction, Intrapsychic Conflict, Interpersonal Violence, edited by Eli Coleman, PhD, S. Margretta Dwyer, MA, and Nathaniel J. Pallone, PhD (Vol. 23, No. 3/4, 1996). *"Offers a review of current assessment and treatment theory while addressing critical issues such as standards of care, use of phallometry, and working with specialized populations such as exhibitionists and developmentally disabled clients. . . . A valuable addition to the reader's professional library." (Robert E. Freeman-Longo, MRC, LPC, Director, The Safer Society Press)*

The Psychobiology of Aggression: Engines, Measurement, Control, edited by Marc Hillbrand, PhD, and Nathaniel J. Pallone, PhD (Vol. 21, No. 3/4, 1995). *"A comprehensive sourcebook for the increasing dialogue between psychobiologists, neuropsychiatrists, and those interested in a full understanding of the dynamics and control of criminal aggression." (Criminal Justice Review)*

Young Victims, Young Offenders: Current Issues in Policy and Treatment, edited by Nathaniel J. Pallone, PhD (Vol. 21, No. 1/2, 1994). *"Extremely practical. . . . Aims to increase knowledge about the patterns of youthful offenders and give help in designing programs of prevention and rehabilitation." (S. Margretta Dwyer, Director of Sex Offender Treatment Program, Department of Family Practice, University of Minnesota)*

Sex Offender Treatment: Psychological and Medical Approaches, edited by Eli Coleman, PhD, S. Margretta Dwyer, and Nathaniel J. Pallone, PhD (Vol. 18, No. 3/4, 1992). *"Summarizes research worldwide on the various approaches to treating sex offenders for both researchers and clinicians." (SciTech Book News)*

The Clinical Treatment of the Criminal Offender in Outpatient Mental Health Settings: New and Emerging Perspectives, edited by Sol Chaneles, PhD, and Nathaniel J. Pallone, PhD (Vol. 15, No. 1, 1990). *"The clinical professional concerned with the outpatient treatment of the criminal offender will find this book informative and useful." (Criminal Justice Review)*

Older Offenders: Current Trends, edited by Sol Chaneles, PhD, and Cathleen Burnett, PhD (Vol. 13, No. 2, 1985). *"Broad in scope and should provide a fruitful beginning for future discussion and exploration." (Criminal Justice Review)*

Prisons and Prisoners: Historical Documents, edited by Sol Chaneles, PhD (Vol. 10, No. 1/2, 1985). *"May help all of us . . . to gain some understanding as to why prisons have resisted change for over 300 years. . . . Very challenging and very disturbing." (Public Offender Counseling Association)*

Gender Issues, Sex Offenses, and Criminal Justice: Current Trends, edited by Sol Chaneles, PhD (Vol. 9, No. 1/2, 1984). *"The contributions of the work will be readily apparent to any reader interested in an interdisciplinary approach to criminology and women's studies." (Criminal Justice Review)*

Current Trends in Correctional Education: Theory and Practice, edited by Sol Chaneles, PhD (Vol. 7, No. 3/4, 1983). *"A laudable presentation of educational issues in relation to corrections." (International Journal of Offender Therapy and Comparative Criminology)*

Counseling Juvenile Offenders in Institutional Settings, edited by Sol Chaneles, PhD (Vol. 6, No. 3, 1983). *"Covers a variety of settings and approaches, from juvenile awareness programs, day care, and vocational rehabilitation to actual incarceration in juvenile and adult institutions. . . . Good coverage of the subject." (Canada's Mental Health)*

Strategies of Intervention with Public Offenders, edited by Sol Chaneles, PhD (Vol. 6, No. 1/2, 1982). *"The information presented is well-organized and should prove useful to the practitioner, the student, or for use in in-service training." (The Police Chief)*

Treating Substance Abusers in Correctional Contexts: New Understandings, New Modalities

Nathaniel J. Pallone
Editor

Treating Substance Abusers in Correctional Contexts: New Understandings, New Modalities has been co-published simultaneously as *Journal of Offender Rehabilitation*, Volume 37, Numbers 3/4 2003.

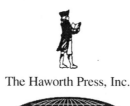

The Haworth Press, Inc.

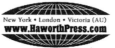

New York • London • Victoria (AU)
www.HaworthPress.com

Treating Substance Abusers in Correctional Contexts: New Understandings, New Modalities has been co-published simultaneously as *Journal of Offender Rehabilitation*™, Volume 37, Numbers 3/4 2003.

Cover design by Brooke R. Stiles

Library of Congress Cataloging-in-Publication Data

Treating substance abusers in correctional contexts : new understandings, new modalities / Nathaniel J. Pallone, editor.
     p. cm.
     "Co-published simultaneously as Journal of offender rehabilitation, volume 37, numbers 3/4 2003."
     Includes bibliographical references and index.
     ISBN 0-7890-2277-X (hard cover : alk. paper) – ISBN 0-7890-2278-8 (soft cover : alk. paper)
     1. Prisoners–Substance use–Prevention. 2. Substance abuse–Treatment. 3. Criminals–Rehabilitation. I. Pallone, Nathaniel J. II. Journal of offender rehabilitation.
HV8836.5.T74 2003
365'.66–dc22   2003017155

Indexing, Abstracting & Website/Internet Coverage

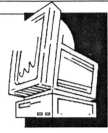

This section provides you with a list of major indexing & abstracting services. That is to say, each service began covering this periodical during the year noted in the right column. Most Websites which are listed below have indicated that they will either post, disseminate, compile, archive, cite or alert their own Website users with research-based content from this work. (This list is as current as the copyright date of this publication.)

Abstracting, Website/Indexing Coverage . . . . Year When Coverage Began

- *CNPIEC Reference Guide: Chinese National Directory of Foreign Periodicals* 1996
- *Contents of this publication are indexed and abstracted in the Social Services PlusText database, available on ProQuest Information & Learning <www.proquest.com>* 1980
- *Criminal Justice Abstracts* 1986
- *Criminal Justice Periodical Index* 1982
- *Environmental Sciences and Pollution Management (Cambridge Scientific Abstracts Internet Database Service) <www.csa.com>* . . . . . . *
- *e-psyche, LLC <www.e-psyche.net>* 1999
- *ERIC Clearinghouse on Counseling and Student Services (ERIC/CASS)* 1983
- *Expanded Academic ASAP <www.galegroup.com>* 1999
- *Expanded Academic ASAP–International <www.galegroup.com>* . . . 1999
- *Family & Society Studies Worldwide <www.nisc.com>* 1996
- *Family Violence & Sexual Assault Bulletin* 1992
- *Gay & Lesbian Abstracts <www.nisc.com>* 2001

(continued)

- *IBZ International Bibliography of Periodical Literature <www.saur.de>* 1996
- *Index Guide to College Journals (core list compiled by integrating 48 indexes frequently used to support undergraduate programs in small to medium sized libraries)* 1999
- *Index to Periodical Articles Related to Law* 1991
- *National Clearinghouse on Child Abuse & Neglect Information Documents Database <www.calib.com/nccanch>* 2001
- *National Criminal Justice Reference Service <www.ncjrs.org>* 1982
- *NIAAA Alcohol and Alcohol Problems Science Database (ETOH) <http://etoh.niaaa.nih.gov>* 1995
- *OCLC ArticleFirst <www.oclc.org/services/databases/>* . . . . *
- *OCLC ContentsFirst <www.oclc.org/services/databases/>* . . . . *
- *OmniFile Full Text: Mega Edition (only available electronically) <www.hwwilson.com>*. 1999
- *Psychological Abstracts (PsycINFO) <www.apa.org>* 1999
- *Referativnyi Zhurnal (Abstracts Journal of the All-Russian Institute of Scientific and Technical Information–in Russian)* . . . 1986
- *Sage Urban Studies Abstracts (SUSA)*. 1992
- *Social Sciences Abstracts & Social Sciences Full Text indexes, abstracts and contains full text to more than 460 publications, specifically selected by librarians and library patrons. <www.hwwilson.com>*. 1999
- *Social Sciences Index (from Volume 1 and continuing) <www.hwwilson.com>*. 1999
- *Social Services Abstracts <www.csa.com>*. 1982
- *Social Work Abstracts <www.silverplatter.com/catalog/swab.htm>*. 1982
- *Sociological Abstracts (SA) <www.csa.com>* 1982
- *Special Educational Needs Abstracts*. 1989
- *Studies on Women Abstracts <www.tandf.co.uk>* 1998
- *SwetsNet <www.swetsnet.com>* 2001
- *Violence and Abuse Abstracts: A Review of Current Literature on Interpersonal Violence (VAA)* 1994
- *Women, Girls & Criminal Justice Newsletter. For subscriptions, write: Civic Research Institute, 4490 Rte. 27, Box 585, Kingston, NJ 08528*. 2002

* **Exact start date to come.**

(continued)

Special Bibliographic Notes related to special journal issues (separates) and indexing/abstracting:

- indexing/abstracting services in this list will also cover material in any "separate" that is co-published simultaneously with Haworth's special thematic journal issue or DocuSerial. Indexing/abstracting usually covers material at the article/chapter level.
- monographic co-editions are intended for either non-subscribers or libraries which intend to purchase a second copy for their circulating collections.
- monographic co-editions are reported to all jobbers/wholesalers/approval plans. The source journal is listed as the "series" to assist the prevention of duplicate purchasing in the same manner utilized for books-in-series.
- to facilitate user/access services all indexing/abstracting services are encouraged to utilize the co-indexing entry note indicated at the bottom of the first page of each article/chapter/contribution.
- this is intended to assist a library user of any reference tool (whether print, electronic, online, or CD-ROM) to locate the monographic version if the library has purchased this version but not a subscription to the source journal.
- individual articles/chapters in any Haworth publication are also available through the Haworth Document Delivery Service (HDDS).

Treating Substance Abusers in Correctional Contexts: New Understandings, New Modalities

CONTENTS

ABOUT THE EDITOR

Nathaniel J. Pallone, PhD, Editor of the *Journal of Offender Rehabilitation,* is University Distinguished Professor (Psychology), Center of Alcohol Studies, Rutgers University, where he previously served as dean and as academic vice president.

Treating Substance Abusers in Correctional Contexts: New Understandings, New Modalities. Pp. xv-xxi.

Editor's Foreword:
Watching History Unfold, Again–or:
Back to the Future?

NATHANIEL J. PALLONE

Rutgers–The State University of New Jersey

ABSTRACT This editor's foreword is a general introduction to a special issue of the *Journal of Offender Rehabilitation* on the theme *Treating Substance Abusers in Correctional Contexts: New Understandings, New Modalities.* Some personal reminiscences are recounted concerning earlier modalities in the rehabilitative treatment of heroin addicts before the introduction of methadone maintenance. *[Article copies available for a fee from The Haworth Document Delivery Service: 1-800-HAWORTH. E-mail address: <docdelivery@ haworthpress.com> Website: <http://www.HaworthPress.com> © 2003 by The Haworth Press, Inc. All rights reserved.]*

KEYWORDS Editor's foreword, substance abuse, treating substance abusers, correctional treatment, Mobilization for Youth, gang norms

One of the more memorable Friday afternoons of my (then-early) professional life was spent on a street corner in the Hell's Gate section of New York City, now largely absorbed by El Barrio, watching history unfold. It was a sultry April in the mid-1960s, with the early humidity that foreshadows the dog days of August. Dick Banks, my former "mentee" and sometime research assistant at the University of Notre Dame, had now, with PhD safely in hand, become a research psychologist at Notre Dame's Center for the Study of Man, with responsibility for operating a field research station located in a storefront off Second Avenue; his principal tasks involved administering a variety of psychological tests to heroin addicts and their non-addicted siblings in order to study conflicts and coping mechanisms. In a reversal of roles that is not uncommon in academia, I–then newly lured to the faculty at NYU, my alma mater, for many reasons, not least of which was the presence there of Isidore Chein, whose *The Road to H* (1964) had only recently been published–had become a sometime assistant to Dick in that research; Dick later went on to a distinguished career at California's Loma Linda University, specializing in marriage and family therapy. I do not know whether the events of that Friday afternoon contributed materially to his decision not to continue to specialize in researching (and treating) drug addiction.

Save for the pioneering work at the U.S. Public Health Service Hospitals in Kentucky and Texas (Ausubel, 1958), albeit with limited patient capacities, and a relative handful of innovative community-based organizations like New York City's Greenwich House and Riverside Hospital (Osnos & Laskowitz, 1966), most members of the mental health and social service communities were, back then, likely to run the other way when confronted with a drug addict, whether on the street or in the waiting room. Although municipal hospitals sometimes provided "drunk tanks" in which the acutely inebriated could attempt to overcome *delirium tremens* during what was typically a maximum stay of three days in a locked ward, little treatment was available for alcoholism either. The brave, new world of the CAC and the CADC, the 28-day residential treatment program (aka "the month in the country"), even the concentration of Federal attention through new agencies like the National Institute on Alcohol Abuse and the National Institute on Drug Abuse, lay years ahead. Indeed, it is perhaps not too much to say that, in those days, the land itself was relatively blind and the one-eyed might readily become, or at least pose as, king.

The conventional wisdom in the mental health sciences held that drug addiction resulted from intrapersonal, psychodynamic forces themselves the product of such underlying psychiatric disorders as "sociopathy" (Robbins, 1966). To the contrary, Chein and his colleagues (1964) had proposed that behavioral contagion and the demographics of communities might have at least as much to do with drug misuse as pre-existing psychopathology–and, even more radically, that perhaps such psychopathology as could be assessed and "post-dicted" among self-identified addicts resulted from, rather than preceded, the addiction itself. As a result of the data gathered at the field research station, Dick and I were able to lend some modest empirical support to such propositions (Pallone & Banks, 1967).

In any case, on the particular afternoon in question, there arose a clatter at the Second Avenue end of the block, and, since we had no scheduled interviews for at least another 30 minutes, we decided to mosey down to have a gawk. What greeted us was an unmarked police car–those were the days of the unmistakable "Kojak-mobile" of television fame–the front seat of which was occupied by two Anglos who seemed to resemble Central Casting's notion of plainclothes police officers. In the back, there sat a single (apparently Hispanic) male, rather obviously in custody. Surrounding the vehicle, there were perhaps 150 residents of the neighborhood, generally expressing their dissatisfaction with the arrest and immobilizing the vehicle, gently rocking it to and fro and absolutely impeding its movement; one of the Anglos was speaking rapidly into the microphone of a car radio. No weapons were in evidence on either side, but there were shouts, moans, and grumbles from the assembled throng.

Dick inquired, in his passable Spanish (acquired during his days as a religious missionary), as to the source of the conflict; after all, it might be the case that we were witnessing an attempted lynching, *a la* New York City, of a notorious serial murderer or rapist. Not so; the police, we were told, had shown the temerity to arrest a person who, in today's argot, would be called the Local Candy Man–and the citizenry didn't like it. His stock in trade was said to be limited marijuana and heroin, with the one representing (once again, in the conventional wisdom) the "gateway" to the other; cocaine and LSD were, back then, "upper middle class" drugs not likely to be found in El Barrio, and we were years away from the development of synthetics like PCP or Angel Dust, the importation of the more exotic forms of cactus or mushroom, the widespread illicit distribution of pharmaceutical preparations with psychoactive properties, the process of crystallizing cocaine into crack.

We had little time to process the scene–that is, both the arrest and the community's response–before there emerged from the next street, on which the local precinct house stood, a detachment of a dozen or so heavily armed police, arrayed in the helmets, goggles, and vests that would become the characteristic battle array of specialized units that were only beginning to be called SWAT teams. As the phalanx turned the corner into Second Avenue, the detachment's commander signaled a halt. Palpably, tension mounted; furiously, the commander and the plainclothes officers appeared to be in conversation, perhaps with each other; then, with a great show of divesting himself of his weapons, the commander approached the car, opened the door, and set the arrestee free. For their part, the assembled citizenry released the sort of satisfied noise Dick and I were accustomed to hear only when Notre Dame scored on its home gridiron against Michigan State or USC.

And then it was over. The crowd dispersed, the SWAT team retreated to the station house, the motor vehicle moved on, unimpeded. In what we even then understood to be a symbolic act, Dick and I turned the corner to go back to the storefront. But we knew that not only the two of us but a rather large and important segment of society had turned another kind of corner, too–that we had witnessed the unfolding of history.

Later on, we attempted as best we could to learn what had motivated the decision to cancel the arrest, to avoid the confrontation, to defuse the pending crisis. Was it perhaps (as today's conspiracy theorist might argue) a case of mistaken identity, in which an early-day Serpico or a police informant had been collared? Or was it merely the case, as we came to believe, that a judgment had been made that the only way to sustain the arrest of the presumed drug dealer would have involved injury (or perhaps death) to one or several of the citizenry who believed the community's interests were not best served by that arrest–that is to say, that keeping the peace took precedence over enforcing the law? If so, at what level was that judgment made–by the SWAT team leader, the watch commander, the precinct captain, the police commissioner, the mayor? No formal answers were forthcoming; nor was the press as dogged in its pursuit of "the whole story" as it has since become.

But it was not the case that the community universally applauded the release of the Candy Man. One resident who derided that decision was a young man in his late 20s whom we knew as Chino. When he first came into contact with us, Chino evinced considerable suspicion toward a couple of Anglos, periodically joined by some Anglo grad students, hanging out in El Barrio and spending a whole lot of time with folk who were fairly obviously drug users, if not addicts. Were we there for a walk on the wild side? To size up a situation so that a drug distributorship could be launched? But the spirit of Notre Dame's "subway alumni" was very much alive and kicking in the New York of that era, so it is likely that the great seal of the University on the front window precluded outright hostility (or worse) on Chino's part and that of a small cadre of like-minded community residents.

Once we were able to convince him that our interests lay in understanding the dynamics of addiction, including the portals and pathways, Chino became a frequent visitor. Yet he was strongly of the opinion that soft-headed approaches such as might be expected of the behavioral and mental health sciences were unlikely to yield usable information. Indeed, he opined that it was precisely such soft-headed approaches that had led to the present infestation of drug use in the city.

A decade earlier, as depicted artistically by Leonard Bernstein in *West Side Story,* street wars between youth gangs were common, with brass knuckles and "Saturday night specials" (sometimes homemade and bearing but a single shot) the weapons of choice (or availability). Though such primitive devices pale in comparison to the firepower in the automatic and semiautomatic weapons wielded by drug-trafficking gangs today, they were nonetheless deadly. A remarkable organization called Mobilization for Youth emerged to address the carnage, in the process creating the "street worker" whose task it was to infiltrate youth gangs and, once accepted as a member, both to attempt to affect group cohesion and to alter group norms. Mobilization had succeeded to the extent that, by the early 1960s, the number of gangs and gang members and the frequency of carnage had indeed receded–albeit that, with some degree of frequency, the Mobilization program is cited as a classic example of the failure to anticipate the consequences of planned intervention in social systems (Helfgot, 1981).

And therein, Chino told us, lay the seeds of the current infestation. For one of the central beliefs common to all gangs, he said, was that every junkie is a s–head. Junkie-whacking had become a common sport among all gangs. Indeed, sometimes rival gangs made common cause by targeting the same junkie or group of junkies for a high old time that yielded more kicks than the prototypical inter-gang rumble. Inter-gang rumbles generally proceeded on the basis of no readily identifiable, tangible, proximate motive; they happened merely because, palpably, an "us" and a "them" could be discerned. But junkie-whacking, whether by one gang or by two or more in concert, arose from a clear norm and a readily discernible motive and, in the bargain, seemed to have all sorts of pro-social benefits. That "we" keep the s–heads out anchored the argument about "our" value to the neighborhood and simultaneously justified "our" resentment against interference, whether by police or these new-fangled "street workers."

On the basis of what we knew about the research in aversive conditioning, Dick and I could scarcely deny that the prospect of being beaten senseless if observed "nodding out" likely served to dissuade at least some drug users from the pursuit of their habit. So, Chino said, if we were genuinely interested in ridding the streets of drugs and drug users, we ought to make it possible for him and a handful of trusted allies to arm themselves, reestablish a network of gangs, and reinstitute the ironclad norm that prized junkie-whacking for the social good. Fortunately (from our perspective), the terms of the research grant under which we were operating permitted no such intervention. Once he understood that, Chino visited us less frequently, instead devoting himself more assiduously to his full-time occupation–collecting debts for street-level loan sharks who calculated interest charges on a daily basis. His instrument of choice in his daily rounds, we had learned, was a lead-filled baseball bat.

Although Chino and like-minded former gang members might stand foursquare for sharply punitive responses to drug use, the dominant societal response adopted legislatively by the state of New York moved sharply away from punishment and in the direction of medicalization and treatment–mirroring, in at least a rough way, the symbolic corner-turning Dick and I had witnessed. In what must surely constitute the most comprehensive public program ever devised to address drug use, the Rockefeller administration shepherded the creation of the New York Narcotics Addiction Control Commission. The Commission had a mandate to seize an arrestee for any offense in which drug use was suspected or otherwise implicated and to commit that arrestee to nine months of residential treatment in a secure (locked) facility, followed by 27 months of "aftercare," initially at least weekly, as constituent elements in a massive pretrial diversion. Successful completion of the rehabilitation program resulted in the expunging of the initial criminal charges, while failure at any point in the 36-month process resulted in incarceration to await trial on those charges–but without credit for "time served," even while "locked in" during residential treatment. During the first seven years of its existence, the Commission treated, with relative success, tens of thousands of drug users (in those days, primarily those habituated to heroin) before its personnel-heavy, mental health-oriented rehabilitation programs gave way to methadone maintenance as an alternative, but substantially less costly, form of (nonetheless) medicalized treatment (Rettig & Yarmolinsky, 1995).

Roughly contemporaneously with the decision in New York to substitute methadone maintenance for the Narcotics Commission's program of psychosocial rehabilitation, "therapeutic nihilism" emerged in the form of the first "Martinson Report" (as the next paper in this volume details more fully). An oscillation away from rehabilitation and toward punitive incarceration in corrections generally had begun, inevitably dictating a return to criminalization as the dominant societal response to drug use and abuse, to be joined to be sure by the gathering momentum of mandatory sentencing legislation for all manner of offenses (drug and otherwise), including those that had earlier been classed as misdemeanors, dictated by the triumph of the "just deserts" perspective not only in penology but in legislative chambers nationwide.

Especially after the establishment of a "drug czar" in the Executive Office of the President during the Reagan administration and the mounting of a "war on drugs" with that officer as its commanding general, criminalization became the centrifugal societal response, with medicalization-rehabilitation in obvious decline but not in total eclipse. Indeed, as the contents of this volume clearly demonstrate, treatment programs for substance users and misusers continued to make significant progress even when not at center stage and–because financial support for the "war on drugs" gave top priority to trammeling the "supply side" (indeed, to the extent of equipping and arming the military of Colombia while simultaneously providing for U.S. military involvement in the aerial surveillance of coca-growing fields)–even though chronically starved financially. Yet, despite the consumption of massive public funds during the past two decades and more (including funds for the construction of prison facilities to house drug users under mandatory sentencing laws), as has been widely documented both in the scholarly journals and in the popular press, neither have the efforts to interdict supply nor the criminalization-punishment axis yielded the anticipated benefits.

The case might be argued that the voters of California in 2000, the Governor of New York a year later, and the drug czar who became "the drug warrior who would rather treat than fight" (as detailed in the next paper) were, in a sense, responding to an idea whose time had come. If these events prove not merely aberrant blips in an otherwise stable criminalize-and-punish, damn-the-torpedoes and full-speed-ahead set of public policies, it is inevitable that we need to look to the past to shape the future. As both policy-makers, legislators, and the professional community begin to reinvent or to retool the medicalization-treatment perspective into a contemporary key, the programs and findings described in this work will provide valuable insights, understandings, signposts, anchors, and seedlings. The scholars and clinicians whose studies are included herein have kept the flame alive.

REFERENCES

Ausubel, D.P. 1958. *Drug Addiction: Physiological, Psychological, and Sociological Aspects.* New York: Random House.

Chein, I., D.L. Gerard, R.S. Lee & B. Rosenfeld. 1964. *The Road to H: Narcotics, Delinquency, and Social Policy.* New York: Basic Books.

Helfgot, J.H. 1981. *Professional Reforming: Mobilization for Youth and the Failure of Social Science.* Lexington, MA: Lexington Books.

Osnos, R., & D. Laskowitz. 1966. *A Counseling Center for Drug Addicts.* New York: Greenwich House. (Available in facsimile through the United Nations Office on Drugs & Crime @ www.undcp.org)

Pallone, N.J., & R.R. Banks. 1967. *High in Hell's Gate: Conflicts and Coping Mechanisms Among Heroin Addicts and Their Non-Addicted Siblings.* Washington: Psychosocial Study Seminar, Vocational Rehabilitation Administration, April.

Retting, R.A., & A. Yarmolinsky. 1995. *Federal Regulation of Methadone Treatment.* Washington: National Academy Press.

Robbins, L. 1966. *Deviant Children Grow Up: A Sociological and Psychiatric Study of Sociopathic Personality.* Baltimore: Williams & Wilkins.

AUTHOR'S NOTE

Nathaniel J. Pallone, PhD, editor-in-chief of the *Journal of Offender Rehabilitation*, is University Distinguished Professor (Psychology), Center of Alcohol Studies, at Rutgers–The State University of New Jersey, where he previously served as dean and as academic vice president. Early in his career, he served for six years as senior consulting psychologist to the New York State Narcotics Addiction Control Commission.

Address correspondence to Dr. N. J. Pallone, 215 Smithers Hall, Center of Alcohol Studies, Rutgers–The State University, New Brunswick, NJ 08901 (E-mail: NJP1800@aol.com).

Treating Substance Abusers in Correctional Contexts: New Understandings, New Modalities. Pp. 1-25.
10.1300/J076v37n03_01

To Punish or to Treat:
Substance Abuse Within the Context
of Oscillating Attitudes
Toward Correctional Rehabilitation

NATHANIEL J. PALLONE

Rutgers–The State University of New Jersey

JAMES J. HENNESSY

Fordham University

ABSTRACT Although its remote origins can be traced to the end of prohibition with the repeal of the Volstead Act in 1933, the nation's "war on
drugs" gathered massive strength in the early days of the Reagan administration. During the 1980s and 1990s, the decision of the nation, expressed
through its legislators, seemed to be to "criminalize" drug use or abuse
through imposition of harsh penalties for what had earlier been statutorily
defined as relatively minor offenses and by eliminating judicial discretion
in sentencing, so that mandatory incarceration was required for many offenses. Yet by 2000, the voters of California, the Governor and criminal
court judges of New York, and even the nation's "drug czar" had decided
that they would rather, as described by the *New York Times*, "treat than
fight." This paper situates that sea change in posture within a context of oscillation toward the goals of corrections generally during an era in which
"therapeutic nihilism" and "just deserts" appeared to have carried the day.
*[Article copies available for a fee from The Haworth Document Delivery Service:
1-800-HAWORTH. E-mail address: <docdelivery@haworthpress.com> Website:
<http://www.HaworthPress.com> © 2003 by The Haworth Press, Inc. All rights
reserved.]*

KEYWORDS Drug abuse, criminal sanctions, therapeutic nihilism, "just deserts," voter rebellion, public policy

To criminalize, or to medicalize–that is, and has been, the question on which societal attitudes toward the use of mood-altering substances of one or another sort have pivoted throughout the 20th century. If substance use, misuse, or abuse be encoded as criminal activity, the appropriate societal response is punishment; but if it be encoded as a medical (or even behavioral) condition (or illness), the appropriate societal response is clearly treatment.

Prohibition of the manufacture and sale of beverage alcohol constituted, of course, the century's grand experiment in criminalization, both in the United States and in many European nations. If Hofmann and Hofmann (1975) are to be believed, wide-scale additions to the roster of "controlled dangerous substances" mandated by the Federal Congress during the 1930s came about at least in part as the consequence of the repeal of the Volstead Act in 1933, thereby rendering obsolete an entire industry that had been organized to police traffic in ethanol. Indeed, it was not until 1975, some 40 years after repeal of the Volstead Act, that alcoholism came to be definitively categorized, by act of Congress, no less, as a disease rather than as a "voluntary misbehavior" (Fingarette, 1988, 1990), albeit as an afterthought in an amendment to legislation concerning vocational rehabilitation–and a new industry was thereby born. But even as new professions (e.g., "certified alcoholism counselor") and new institutions (rehabilitation centers, typically offering a 28-day residential treatment program) were generated, however, public inebriation remained a crime in most jurisdictions.

If the Hofmanns' rendition seems too cynical a reading, yet it should be noted that, as this paper is written, the popular press has widely reported results of a RAND study that sharply counters the conventional wisdom that use of marijuana places one on the slippery slope that leads only to depravity, a finding that appears to support the *Wall Street Journal's* famous (or infamous, depending upon one's cherished beliefs) characterization of US drug laws as "the criminalization of the common pleasures of the underclasses." Indeed, the RAND Corporation's public affairs office (2002) itself asserted in a press release that results of the study "challenge an assumption that has guided US drug policies since the 1950s."

The nation's "war on drugs" dates, under that specific rubric, from the early days of the Reagan administration. It is a fair assessment to say that, during the 1980s and 1990s, criminalization of substance abuse constituted the dominant theme, so that laws governing the use, sale, importation, or manufacture of an ever-expanding litany of "controlled dangerous substances" (and their "workalike" counterparts, whether obtained by prescription or even "over the counter") were strengthened, with formal sanctions either attached thereto or rendered more severe. Making sanctions more severe included in some instances legislatively mandating incarceration for offenses that either had not been earlier classified as felonies or in the imposition of penalty in situations in which there had previously been wide judicial latitude.

But at the cusp of the millennium there were strong indications on both ocean coasts of the nation that a tectonic shift had begun, yielding a situation in which, according to the *New York Times* (Wren, 2001), playing on the phrasing of a once-popular television commercial urging brand loyalty in the consumption of tobacco, even the nation's "drug czar" had decided that he "would rather treat than fight." It is the purpose of this paper to situate that emergent shift within the context of oscillation in societal attitudes and perceptions about who should be "punished" and who should be "treated" within, or under the aegis of, a correctional "system" comprised both of penal institutions and community agencies and resources.

SCOPE OF THE CORRECTIONAL "SYSTEM"

Official records of the Bureau of Justice Statistics, the agency of the US Department of Justice with responsibility for collating data of all sorts concerning the criminal justice system, suggest that some 5.7 million people were (to use the term current in Federal parlance) "under correctional supervision" (Maguire & Pastore, 1999, 462), distributed among prisons, jails, and parole and probation agencies (as depicted in Figure 1) during a single year near the end of the twentieth century. Those given to this sort of thing might want to observe that, in the aggregate, slightly more than 2% of the nation's population of 280 million were thus "under correctional supervision" during the year in review.

Offenders under "community supervision" on probation or parole comprise nearly 70% of the total, outnumbering offenders incarcerated in state or Federal prisons as a result of felony convictions at a ratio greater than 3:1 and outnumbering the population of jails (composed of both accused offenders awaiting trial or the posting of bail and of convicted misdemeanants) at a ratio greater than 7:1. The matter of the type of facility in which offenders are held (prisons, with relatively stable populations serving sentences of specified lengths, vs. jails, with their revolving door clientele) and for how long represent important variables in the planning and delivery of medical, psychosocial, mental health, or other "treatment" services.

In general, psychosocial, treatment services are provided to incarcerated offenders by employees of the correctional authority (i.e., state, county, or Federal department of corrections), although a trend has emerged toward the "privatization" of many such services (Demone & Gibelman, 1990; Bowman, Hakim & Seidenstat, 1993; Kronick, 1993) in much the same way that correctional institutions have long contracted with private vendors to operate food preparation services. In either case, the character (and sometimes the fre-

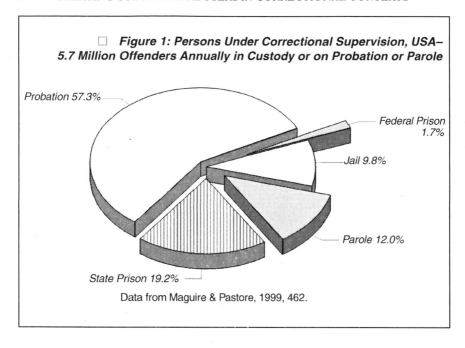

☐ **Figure 1: Persons Under Correctional Supervision, USA–**
5.7 Million Offenders Annually in Custody or on Probation or Parole

Probation 57.3%

Federal Prison
1.7%

Jail 9.8%

Parole 12.0%

State Prison 19.2%

Data from Maguire & Pastore, 1999, 462.

quency) of treatment and/or rehabilitation services is determined by policies of the correctional authority, in their turn responsive to legislative and judicial instruction. In contrast, offenders under community supervision are usually served by social service or mental health agencies in the community whose policies are not controlled by the correctional authority. Generally, direct referral to relevant community agencies (including outpatient clinics at hospitals) is made by the probation or parole officer; less frequently, referral is made to community agencies or institutions under contractual relationships to serve offender clients.

It is a matter of more than passing interest that whites, who constituted 80% of the nation's population in the 2000 census, comprise only 60% of the correctional population depicted in Figure 1. Similarly, according to the 2000 census, girls and women constituted 51% of the general population, but they represent only 16% of the correctional population. Demographic disparities between the population in general and the offender population clearly impinge upon the planning and delivery of correctional rehabilitation services.

OSCILLATING ATTITUDES TOWARD CORRECTIONS

At least since the time of the Marquis di Beccaria in the 18th century, the goals of corrections have been conceded to include *incapacitation, retribution,* deterrence, and *rehabilitation* (Taylor & Brasswell, 1979; Welch, 1999), generally within the context of the principle of *proportionality* between offense and sanction traceable to the Code of Hammurabi in the 18th century BC and reinforced in the British Magna Carta three millennia later. In response to societal, political, and intellectual forces (Foucault, 1978), emphasis has of course shifted among and between these four goals over time, so that one or the other, or some permutation, may temporarily discernibly ascend and others recede.

Penance vs. Punishment: Rehabilitation as an American Tradition

Indeed, an oscillation of substantial proportions occurred not long after the founding of the American republic, when in 1787 the Quakers of Pennsylvania invented the *penitentiary* as an alternative to the *prison*, the purpose of which had historically been to punish and incapacitate. In contrast, the Quaker penitentiary was to be a place where offenders were confined to do penance through religious meditation and "spiritual exercises" and thus become "penitent" for their transgressions, in the process vowing irrevocably, with the aid of the Almighty, to forego wrongdoing forevermore.

However much the religious-spiritual dimension which shaped the Quaker invention may have eroded, there is little question that, half a century ago, if rehabilitation did not quite stand univocally as the primary goal of corrections (Lindner, 1949; American Friends Service Committee, 1971), it surely stood alongside incapacitation, deterrence, and retribution as *primus inter pares*. Legislators and the general public alike expected, and were willing to finance, the provision of rehabilitation services of various sorts for offenders incarcerated in the nation's prisons and, sometimes, jails.

Pugh v. Locke: *The Right of Prison Inmates to Mental Health "Care"*

A perception of rehabilitation as a primary purpose in corrections is readily inferrable in the landmark 1976 decision of Federal appellate court judge Frank M. Johnson in *Pugh v. Locke*, a case concerning the operation of the prisons of Alabama, later upheld by the US Supreme Court and, therefore, uniformly precedental throughout the nation. In his decision, Mr. Johnson imposed a wide-ranging set of "minimum Constitutional standards for inmates" that mandated "humane" and sanitary living conditions (with strict standards imposed to address prison overcrowding), "meaningful programs" staffed by qualified personnel, and at least first-line mental health care within correctional institutions (Fowler, 1976, 1987). Over the next two decades, no fewer than 37 states were ordered by the Federal courts to meet the standards specified in *Pugh*.

Federal courts in the southern tier had earlier issued the linchpin decisions in *Donaldson v. O'Connor*, *Wyatt v. Hardin,* and *Wyatt v. Stickney*, cases brought on behalf of patients confined in public mental hospitals. In upholding those decisions, the US Supreme Court declared unequivocally that patients in mental hospitals have an absolute *right to treatment* and that to confine patients in the absence of treatment in effect constitutes involuntary imprisonment, in violation of the Constitutional guarantees against deprivation of liberty without due process contained in the 8th and 14th Amendments (Golann & Fremouw, 1976, 129-185).

But, although he affirmed the right of inmates to mental health *care*, Mr. Johnson stopped far short in *Pugh* of articulating a right to *treatment*. Instead, he ordered that prison administrators "shall identify those inmates who require mental health care within the institution and make arrangements for such care," while simultaneously ordering that there should be "routine" provision for identification of "those inmates who, by reason of psychological disturbance or mental retardation require care in facilities designed for such persons" and for the transfer of prisoners thus identified to such (presumably forensic) psychiatric installations. From the judicial perspective, "treatment" thus appears to be that form of professional intervention provided in psychiatric hospitals, while "care" is that form of intervention to be provided *in situ* for prisoners whose disorders are not severe enough to warrant hospitalization. Although it has been at pains in its *Diagnostic and Statistical Manual of Mental Disorders, Fourth Edition* to label an enormous array of human behaviors–including, indeed, a singular devotion to soft drinks that contain caffeine–as psychopathological, the psychiatric community has rather anomalously not chosen to quarrel with those distinctions, implicitly ceding the *in situ* treatment of offenders to non-psychiatrists (Schnapp & Cannedy, 1998; Badger, Vaughn, Woodward & Williams, 1999).

Pugh specifically adopts the mental health staffing ratios proposed by the Center for Correctional Psychology at the University of Alabama (Gormally, Brodsky, Clements & Fowler, 1972), which reduce to an overall ratio of one mental health specialist for each 91 inmates–specifically: one bachelor's level mental health technician or correctional counselor for each 135 inmates; one psychologist for each 506 inmates; one social worker for each 578 inmates; one psychiatrist for each 4,048 inmates. Mr. Johnson's ruling in effect held that these personnel were required to provide "mental health care" as a sort of first-line intervention within the prisons themselves, since the most severe cases were to be transferred to appropriate mental hospital facilities. It might be noted that inventories of mental health staffing in state prisons shortly after *Pugh* provided evidence of enormous discrepancies between those standards, staff actually employed and deployed, and staffing standards promulgated by such organizations as the American Correctional Association (Pallone & LaRosa, 1979; Pallone, Hennessy & LaRosa, 1980). In a similar context, at least one legal scholar (Mayer, 1990) has labeled the failure of correctional administrators to meet court-imposed standards an exemplar of Constitutionally impermissible "deliberate indifference." And, in view of the definitive *Pugh* standards governing prison overcrowding, it is distressing to observe that, nearly a quarter century after that historic decision, the number of prisoners held in correctional institutions exceeded the capacity of those institutions by 25% in the Federal system, 72% in California, 77% in Hawaii, 41% in Illinois, 20% in Indiana, 64% in Iowa, an astounding 230% in Massachusetts, 96% in Montana, 39% in Nebraska, 46% in New Jersey, 69% in Ohio, 51% in Pennsylvania, 55% in Virginia, 41% in Washington, and 48% in Wisconsin (Maguire & Pastore, 1999, 487). That the prison systems of 14 states, including several major population centers, and the Federal system itself apparently no longer perceive themselves bound by the "minimum Constitutional standards" enunciated in *Pugh* perhaps reveals a posture for which "deliberate indifference" may be too euphemistic a descriptor.

Martinson, "Nothing Works," and the Seeds of Therapeutic Nihilism

However favorable to rehabilitation the prevailing ethos then seemed to be, countervailing forces were at work. Even the entertainment media entered the lists, with offender rehabilitation parodied mercilessly by director Stanley Kubrick in his 1971 film version of Anthony Burgess' *A Clockwork Orange*. With the publication of the now-famous (or perhaps infamous) Martinson Report, empirical challenges were directly mounted against the primacy of rehabilitation as a goal in corrections. Media attention immediately surrounded publication of Martinson's report on the efficacy of rehabilitation efforts in prisons (1974) largely because the government agency which had sponsored the study on which the report was based had formally suppressed its release.

In 1971, a major prisoner revolt had taken place at the New York state prison at Attica, ultimately claiming 43 lives. Among the "non-negotiable" demands made by leaders of the revolt were requests for increased quantity and quality in rehabilitation services; as Governor of the state, Nelson Rockefeller quickly agreed. However, there was underway at the time a major study of the effectiveness of rehabilitation programs of all sorts in correctional institutions of various sorts. Because its conclusions countered the state's capitulation to prisoners' demands, and because it constituted a "work for hire" and could thus quite legitimately be classified as "confidential," state administrators ordered that no report of the research be released. But the leaders of the revolt knew of the study and of Martinson's role as an investigator (though not the principal investigator). At their trial on varied criminal charges, they sought to mitigate responsibility by appealing to the evidence accumulated by the research team that showed rehabilitation to be relatively ineffective. The research saw the light of day only when the judge presiding in those trials ordered that the suppression be lifted. Thus it was that the "Martinson Report" (1974), published in the neo-conservative "journal of opinion" *The Public Interest* rather than in a peer-reviewed scholarly journal in the behavioral sciences, became almost instantly a focus of national press attention.

Martinson concluded that most offender rehabilitation regimens for adult prisoners constitute a colossal waste of professional energy and of taxpayers' money. That dire judgment was mollified somewhat in a more detailed monograph by Lipton, Martinson and Wilks (1975)–and indeed mollified even further by Lipton (1995), the lead investigator, in a 20-year retrospective in the pages of this journal. But a similarly pessimistic conclusion was reached by Shamsie (1981) in an ambitious review of the research evidence on the effectiveness of similar rehabilitation efforts among juvenile offenders. Predictably, members of the professional community committed to rehabilitation as a governing purpose of corrections sought to answer the Martinson judgments (Cullen & Gilbert, 1982; Gendreau & Ross, 1979; Glaser, 1979), often with more heat than light. As Martinson (1976) himself suggested, these responses may have issued from a sense of disbelief that "all the well-intentioned efforts of the psychiatric, psychological, and social service communities, of the medical establishment, of the prisons and the jails, and even of the schools have yielded such disappointing results."

The controversy reached even into the prestigious National Academy of Sciences, which commissioned a blue-ribbon panel to reanalyze the more than 200 studies of rehabilitation effectiveness on which the Lipton, Martinson and Wilks conclusions were based (Sechrest, White & Brown, 1979). Those excruciating reanalyses (Feinberg & Gramsbach, 1979) did little to alter the "gloomy conclusions" reached by Martinson, even though (in what may have been more a leap of faith than a reasoned scientific judgment) Sechrest, White and Brown, (1979, 34) focussed on flaws in the research design of the 200-plus studies which had yielded those negative conclusions: "The quality of the work that has been done . . . militate[s] against any policy reflecting a final pessimism." Further reanalyses in Britain of the original data base (Hollin, 1990) similarly focused on the adequacy of the research design employed in the studies represented therein, but, like the National Academy of Science review, declined to draw any sharp conclusion, whether positive or negative. In Hollin's (1990, 119-120) account:

> The ambiguity in clinical outcome studies has been used in both the United Kingdom and the United States to fuel the doctrine maintaining that "nothing works"; that is, any attempt at rehabilitation is doomed to failure. . . . This research is often quoted by those in favor of therapeutic nihilism . . . [yet] the small number of acceptable studies immediately limits the data base from which any conclusions can be drawn, and the subject matter of these studies allows no conclusions to be made. . . .

Enter Meta-Analysis and Aptitude-Treatment Interaction

Chastened though it may have been, offender rehabilitation did not quite pass quietly into the dark night. Contemporaneously, the mental health and social service professions in general had begun to abandon the one-size-fits-all mindset that had once served as its anchor. Instead, great attention began to be paid to "aptitude-treatment interactions." When treatment modalities were "customized" or differentiated for clients or patients with essentially similar "presenting problems," with the customization geared to the characteristics of the individual, positive results seemed to ensue more dependably. A "disorder-aptitude-treatment interaction" approach (or "differential treatment model") began, rather tentatively and perhaps stealthily, to be applied initially to criminal offenders in the community, then in institutions. Results were, in some cases, positive.

It also happened that, shortly after the National Academy's re-review of the Lipton-Martinson-Wilks data, Smith, Glass and Miller (1980) published a monograph promoting a methodology for analyzing the effects of psychotherapy called "meta-analysis." Utilizing relatively high-powered statistical techniques, meta-analysis facilitates the aggregation of data from studies that at first blush seem difficult to compare because they had used variant means of measuring outcomes, varying lengths of time after the termination of treatment before "outcome" was measured, and so on. Two decades after the appearance of the Martinson Report, and indeed during an era that had largely abandoned rehabilitation as the focal service in corrections, evidence began to emerge from studies utilizing the techniques of meta-analysis that to the bald "nothing works" formulation of the 1970s could quite properly be juxtaposed the proposition that *"some things work for some offenders under certain conditions"* (Gendreau & Andrews, 1990; Loesel, 1993, 1995; Hollin, 1999; Redondo, Sanchez-Meca & Garrido, 1999), a proposition that essentially restates the disorder-aptitude-treatment interaction," or "differential treatment" model.

From "Just Deserts" to "Get Tough, Hang 'em High"– and the War on Drugs

At least to some extent fueled by empirical challenges to rehabilitation as a goal in corrections, conceptual challenges were launched by advocates of a "just deserts" policy (Morris, 1974; von Hirsch, 1976, 1984, 1985, 1988; Allen, 1981), who argued that how society deals with an adjudicated offender should follow precisely sanctions prescribed in the criminal code for the offense or offenses of which he/she has been convicted–so that the sanction is in essence predicated by the character of the offense, not the characteristics of the offender–and by the likelihood that he/she may re-offend, a prospect largely to be determined on the basis of the offender's prior criminal record (Sherman & Hawkins, 1981). Moreover, that sanction should not be mitigated in any way by post-offense, post-conviction considerations like progress in a program of rehabilitation.

Accordingly, particularly since early release on parole had become in practice at least related to, if not contingent on, participation in such rehabilitation programs, "just deserts" advocates also sought to curtail sharply parole eligibility. Such eligibility should pivot on completion of a mandatory and inflexible minimum proportion of the sentence imposed. As a codicil, a "just deserts" model quite logically holds that, if psychosocial rehabilitation in the correctional setting had proved dependably effective, its advantages should have been abundantly clear without the protection of equivocal statements about whether valid conclusions can or cannot be drawn from the body of evidence by resorting to the recondite modes of number-crunching demanded by meta-analysis, in feverish efforts to ferret out whatever small statistical advantages may lie therein. Explicitly, then, the "just deserts" model contends that correctional institutions should (once and for all) redefine themselves as places whose purposes are to deter and incapacitate–in short, to punish in precise and inflexible fashion.

"Just deserts" policies found substantial support in the Federal Congress. In a series of measures enacted with bipartisan support–epitomized by the Criminal Sentencing Reform Act (CSRA) of 1981, cosponsored in the Senate by Ted Kennedy and Strom Thurmond, as unlikely a pair of political bedfellows as can be imagined–the Congress embraced a "get tough, hang 'em high" posture toward the Federal correctional system. The pivots in the 1981 Act required

- that sentences to incarceration be rendered mandatory for offenders convicted of certain offenses, thus removing substantial discretion in sentencing previously ceded to judges; and
- that an offender serve a "mandatory minimum" portion of his/her sentence before becoming eligible for parole.

Since Federal prisoners constitute but a small minority of the correctional population of the nation, the 1981 Act directly affected only a tiny proportion of offenders under correctional supervision. But Federal legislation achieves its principal effects indirectly, by rippling outward through widespread imitation by the legislatures of the individual states.

In 1986, Congress enacted the Omnibus Crime Reduction Act (OCRA) as a cornerstone in the Reagan Administration's War on Drugs. OCRA mandates incarceration for a variety of offenses related to the sale or possession of drugs ("controlled dangerous substances," in the Federal lexicon) or of "drug paraphernalia," the penalties for many of which had previously been left to the discretion of judges. Once again, as the "hang 'em high" bandwagon coursed through the nation, OCRA elicited wide imitation by the states.

The direct impact of CSRA and OCRA (and surrounding and supporting legislation) on the Federal prison system can be gauged fairly precisely by considering the data reported by the Bureau of Justice Statistics (Maguire & Pastore, 1999, 505) concerning drug offenders in Federal prison as a proportion of all Federal prisoners. In 1980, before either CSRA or OCRA, there were slightly more than 19,000 Federal prisoners, of whom 25% (4,749) were drug offenders. In 1990, nine years after CSRA and four years after OCRA, the total Federal prison population had more than doubled to 47,000, with 52% (25,000) drug offenders. Within the space of a single decade, during which the general population had increased by only 10% (from 226 to 248 million), the number of Federal prisoners had increased by nearly 150%, or at a rate approximately fifteen times as great as the increase in the general population. Indeed, by 1990 there were 52% more drug offenders incarcerated than the total number of inmates in Federal prisons for any and all offenses ten years earlier. By 1998, the comparisons yielded even greater drama, with a total of 95,000 inmates, including 56,000 (57%) drug offenders. Thus, the number of drug offenders confined in Federal prisons in 1998 was very nearly treble the total number of offenders serving sentences in Federal prisons for any and all offenses in 1970. These data are depicted graphically in Figure 2.

In the prisons of the states, 20% were serving sentences for drug offenses in 1999 (Beck, 2000). In addition, slightly under 10% were serving sentences for a catch-all category called "public order offenses," under which are subsumed "drunk driving" and "liquor law violations." But some investigators have put the proportion of prisoners in state institutions with "diagnosable substance abuse or dependence disorders" as high as 74% (Peters, Greenbaum, Edens, Carter & Ortiz, 1998), even though the instant offense may involve neither alcohol nor drugs directly.

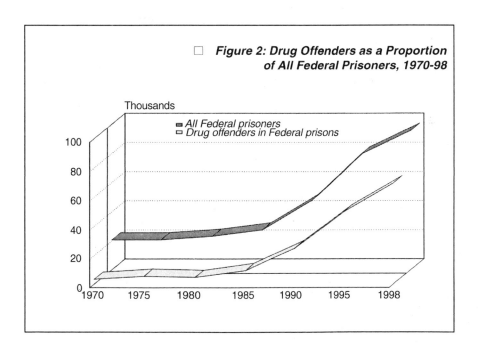

Figure 2: Drug Offenders as a Proportion of All Federal Prisoners, 1970-98

Whether as a function of a "just deserts" sentencing policy in general or of the mandatory sentencing of drug offenders in particular, the growth curve in the state prisons essentially replicates that in the Federal prisons. In 1980, there were 130 state prisoners per 100,000 of the general population (Maguire & Pastore, 1999, 491). By 1990, that rate had increased to 272 per 100,000 (approximately 110%) and, by 1998, to 415 per 100,000 (approximately 220%).

Although it primarily targets adult offenders, a "get tough, hang 'em high" posture extends to juvenile offenders as well, primarily by rendering certain offenses committed by juveniles at some ages (e.g., between 14 and 18) or at any age liable to prosecution and sanctioning under the adult, rather than under the more lenient juvenile, criminal code (Clement, 1997-a; Feld, 1998; Zimring, 1998; Kempf-Leonard & Peterson, 2000).

A "Just Deserts" Perspective on Mental Health Care vs. Rehabilitation

There is no more articulate spokesperson for the "just deserts" perspective than the distinguished legal scholar and criminologist Norval Morris. Even as "just deserts" activists contended vigorously to redefine the prison in particular and corrections more generally, Morris (1974, 14-15) drew capital distinctions between mental health care *as a health service* for confined offenders and mental health care as a component in a program of psychosocial rehabilitation for those conditions thought to be "causative" of criminal behavior:

> "Rehabilitation," whatever it means and whatever the program that allegedly gives it meaning, must cease to be a purpose of the prison sanction. This does *not* mean that the various . . . treatment programs within prisons need to be abandoned; quite the contrary, they need expansion. But it does mean that they must not be seen as *purposive* in the sense that criminals are to be sent to prison *for* treatment. . . . The system is corrupted when we fail to preserve this distinction and this failure pervades the world's prison programs.

From that perspective, the terms of the debate about the primacy of punishment vs. rehabilitation seem not so much wrong-headed as wrong-ended. To regard mental health care as the *purpose* of imprisonment requires an unswerving conviction supported by strong empirical evidence that criminal behavior is the consequence of mental disorder. Hence, once the source disorder is remedied, the criminal behavior can be expected to cease. From comparison of epidemiological studies in the community, in mental hospitals, and in prisons, there is evidence that the relative incidence of mental disorder of any and all diagnosable sort (including "antisocial personality disorder," virtually the defining diagnosis among at least persistent criminal offenders) is greater among prison inmates than in the general population–but not as great as that among mental hospital patients with respect to psychosis, virtually the defining diagnosis among at least repetitively-admitted mental patients (Pallone, 1991). But there is very scant evidence to support the conjecture that criminal behavior is, *therefore,* a function of remediable mental disorder of the same sort as that which characterizes mental hospital patients (Pallone & Hennessy, 1996, 1-20). Within the present context, that is perhaps another way of saying that, if a drug-dependent burglar is "cured" of his/her drug dependence, it is equally plausible to believe that he/she will thereafter become a more efficient burglar since consciousness will no longer be clouded *as it is* to believe that, because he/she no longer needs to support an expensive drug habit, he/she will thereafter become a model citizen.

TO THE DRUG WARRIOR
WHO WOULD RATHER TREAT THAN FIGHT

It is generally estimated that the annual cost of maintenance for a prisoner ranges between $42,000 and $55,000. For a fully informed and informative estimate, however, to that maintenance cost should be added the amortization costs incurred in constructing and equipping prison facilities, which may add another $15,000 to $45,000 per prisoner. However much it satisfies a primordial surge at the visceral level toward vengeance, a "get tough, hang 'em high" policy clearly imposes huge financial burdens upon the taxpayer; and therein lies one of the principal seeds of the Rebellion of 2000.

The taxpayers' contribution to that Rebellion is best exemplified by the adoption of Proposition 36 by the voters of California, the most populous state in the union. As earlier observed, its prison system, operating at 172% capacity, had become hopelessly overcrowded, with a large proportion of inmates serving mandatory sentences for possession of controlled dangerous substances in quantities large enough to suggest nothing more sinister than personal (sometimes called rather too euphemistically termed "recreational") use. Serious doubts had already been expressed as to whether punishment represents an optimal societal response to such offenses (Wexler, Blackmore & Lipton, 1991; Lipton, 1994). The key provision in Proposition 36 repeals the mandatory sentencing provisions of relevant statutes, with the expectation that those guilty of drug possession will instead be placed on probation but required to undergo treatment in the community, whether at the offender's expense or at public expense. Proponents of Proposition 36 emphasized that, even were they to be borne by the public treasury, the annual per-person cost for outpatient treatment for drug use would require far less in cash outlay than current per-prisoner maintenance costs. Moreover, at least some proportion of drug offenders sanctioned in this way could be expected to maintain employment and continue to pay taxes, thus adding to–rather than depleting–the public treasury; and, finally, in some proportions of the cases, the costs of outpatient treatment might be borne by third-party medical insurers or health maintenance organizations rather than the public treasury.

The perceptions and attitudes that motivated rebellion among a cadre of criminal court judges in New York were less well articulated, at least to the public press. Instead, these judges declared themselves essentially to be on strike, asserting that they would hear no further cases involving drug offenses for which incarceration is legislatively mandated *until the state made provision for alternate, community-based drug treatment*, whether through the by-then burgeoning Federally-financed "drug courts" that provide pretrial diversion (Peters & Murrin, 2000; Hennessy, 2001) or elsewise.

Some commentators saw in the declaration by the judges a prospective re-birth of the pretrial intervention strategies (Matthews, 1980) pioneered in the early 1960s by the New York State Narcotics Addiction Control Commission (and imitated elsewhere) under the Rockefeller gubernatorial administration, through which criminal charges lodged against a accused offender who is demonstrably drug-involved are held in abeyance until he/she has completed a course of treatment for addiction, in much the same fashion in which first-time DWI offenders are dealt with in traffic courts (Lucker & Osti, 1997). If treatment is successful, criminal charges are dropped. In the 1960s version, treatment was typically provided under the auspices of a correctional agency in a "secure" facility analogous to a locked forensic psychiatric hospital through long-term inpatient (nine-month) care and outpatient (27-month) aftercare, but the current version appears to favor shorter-term outpatient treatment in the community or even inpatient treatment in a "civilian" rather than "correctional" facility (Jenkins, 1995; Rose, 1997; Peters & Hills, 1999; Hennessy, 2001).

Another variation pursued with vigor in "drug courts" in some jurisdictions interposes treatment between conviction (typically, by virtue of a guilty plea) and sentence. If the drug-involved offender completes treatment satisfactorily and further maintains a drug-free lifestyle for a specified period thereafter (e.g., 12 months), the record of conviction is purged. But if the offender leaves treatment prematurely, he/she is immediately incarcerated to serve the custodial sentence for the offense to which he/she has pled guilty (or of which he/she has been convicted).

As if in response to the threat by the criminal court judges, the Republican Governor of New York proposed in mid-January 2001 a tripartite change in the way in which that state deals with illicit drug use. The key elements in the Governor's plan (Perez-Pena, 2001) provided for

- "shorter prison terms for . . . nonviolent drug offenses,"
- "replacing mandatory imprisonment with treatment," and
- "giving judges greater discretion in handling drug-related criminal charges"

Given the enormous aggregate population of California and New York, accounting for nearly 25% of the nation's total, there seemed little question that what had started life as a taxpayers' rebellion had rather rapidly given rise to a major change in policy with substantial implications for rehabilitation services for offenders both in the community and within correctional institutions.

These developments on the two coasts may represent but minor tremors in an otherwise placid landscape. Alternately, however, the Governor and the criminal court judges of New York and the voters of California may instead be the heralds of yet another oscillation, with rehabilitation once again in ascendancy. That such an interpretation is not woefully off the mark is nowhere better illustrated than in what was widely perceived as a wholesale change in strategy toward substance use and abuse proposed in the waning days of the Clinton Administration by Gen. Barry McCaffrey, then serving as the nation's "drug czar." McCaffrey had presided over a "war on drugs" with its genesis in the early days of the Reagan presidency. The governing policies of the "war on drugs" placed its greatest emphases

- on the "supply" side, on the interdiction of controlled dangerous substances at points of origin (replete with American paratroopers conducting raids on coca growing fields in Colombia and US aircraft and patrol boats assiduously guarding the nation's permeable borders), and
- on the "demand" side, on the punitive incarceration of substance users in American prisons.

But, as he prepared to leave office, Gen. McCaffrey recommended that emphasis shift emphatically to prevention and treatment. The war on drugs, he proposed, should be supplanted by a "crusade against drugs." In a published account of his unexpected conversion, *New York Times* writer Christopher Wren (2001) described McCaffrey as "the drug warrior who would rather treat than fight."

It should not escape notice that the pendulum began to swing not as the result of an emergent flood tide of sentiment favoring humanitarian values over punitive postures, nor even on the basis of a philosophic premise that society has little right to regulate what people ingest, whatever the psychoactive and social consequences (Szasz, 1992; Nadelman, 1993), so that *neither* criminalization *nor* medicalization constitutes an appropriate societal response to substance use. Instead, the pendulum swing seems to have been motivated largely by financial considerations in relation to the relative ineffectiveness of punitive measures (Baum, 1991). Implicitly, the newly-emerging focus (truly, re-focus) on rehabilitation for drug offenders–that is to say, a preference for medicalizing rather than criminalizing–recognizes that punitive incarceration has simply failed either to halt the "epidemic" of drug use/abuse or to reduce recidivism following release from confinement, a position that echoes the long-standing conviction in the literature on penology that prisons are themselves schools for the perfection of the skills associated with crime and hardly harbors for their extirpation (Pallone, 1991; *see also* Hughes, this issue). Nor, moreover, should it escape notice that countervailing arguments favoring the *status quo* are being set forth both by "true believers" and by the "privateers" who operate prison facilities in some states and/or provide staff in other states and who thus stand at risk financially should medicalization once again become dominant in such fashion that the clinic replaces the prison as the principal venue. Such arguments will continue to be propounded at least until it becomes evident to the corporate sponsors of those privateers (and the lobbyists who represent them) that privatization of outpatient drug treatment facilities (especially residential facilities)–to be sure, under contract to state authorities and thus funded through the public treasury–represents fertile but as yet unplowed territory.

CURRENT MODALITIES
IN THE CORRECTIONAL TREATMENT OF DRUG ABUSERS

Even though criminalization, "just deserts," and "get tough" sounded the theme songs of the 1980s and 1990s, treatment and/or rehabilitation services were nonetheless offered in a variety of configurations within correctional institutions and in the community for court-referred or -involved clients. Indeed, the Federal government's Substance Abuse and Mental Health Services Administration (2000) reported that, in a recent year, some 480,000 persons had been served in drug abuse treatment facilities nationwide. That very large total number includes the self-referred as well as those who have mis-used (or have self-identified as having mis-used) either prescription drugs or over-the-counter pharmaceutical preparations, so no assumption can be made about the proportion of the total properly classifiable as "drug offenders."

"Service" might, for example, consist of a single session in which information is provided concerning meetings of self-help groups, whether for the inquirer or a friend or a relative. For clients referred through criminal justice channels, "treatment" might range from brief psychodidactic sessions in consequence of a "driving under the influence" warning to residential treatment programs in the community or within correctional facilities.

Modalities in use in the treatment of substance abusers under the aegis of the correctional system are sometimes modeled after the principles of "rational recovery" (Trimpey, 1996) but more often follow the *"Twelve Step" model* pioneered by the Alcoholics Anonymous movement and adopted by Narcotics Anonymous and, with somewhat lesser relevance, by Gamblers Anonymous and Sex Offenders Anonymous (Cotte, 1997; Anderson, 1999; Wildman, 2000). Treatment patterned after, or incorporating, the Twelve-Step model has been provided for offenders sometimes within correctional settings and sometimes, for probationers and parolees, in the community (Glatt, 1974; Brown,

1985; Greer, Lawson, Baldwin & Cochrane, 1990; Hirschel & Keny, 1990; Peters, May & Kearns, 1992; Scarpiti, Inciardi & Pottieger, 1993; Peters, Kearns, Murrin, Dolente & May, 1993; Wagoner & Piazza, 1993; Tims, Inciardi, Fletcher & Horton, 1997; Ronel, 1998). Direct treatment has in some instances also been provided when needed for family members (McGaha, 1993).

Although he examined only a sample of states and the Federal prison system, Lipton's (1998) review of effectiveness data shows generally positive results for such intervention provided within correctional institutions; Peters and Hills (1999) reached similar conclusions in their review of data from programs in community settings.

In addition to the Twelve-Step model anchored in "talk therapy," alternate and supplemental interventions have included *psychodidactic components* (Newbern, Danserau & Dees, 1997) to educate offenders about the biochemical effects of habituation to substances of various sorts and covert measures for *sensitization and desensitization* (Daniel & Dodd, 1990). In "last chance" cases that have proven refractory to milder treatment and in which life is imminently threatened, *pharmacotherapy* with substance-specific chemical antagonists (e.g., Antabuse in the case of alcohol addiction) has been medically prescribed (Karper, Bennett, Erdos & Krystal, 1994). However, it is a fair assessment to say that, within the correctional community, Twelve-Step programs are prized for their strong emphasis upon self-help and upon extension of help to others who have more recently engaged the process of recovery (Scott, Hawkins & Farnsworth, 1994).

Whatever the modality, focus has generally been placed sharply on *relapse prevention* (Knight, Simpson & Danserau, 1994) rather than on the antecedents to addiction or to its past criminal consequences. Special attention has sometimes been given to the differential pathways to addiction pursued by women (Clement, 1997-b). In view of the massive needs for such intervention among correctional clientele, pilot programs have occasionally been undertaken to train probation and parole officers as paraprofessionals to provide substance abuse treatment (Cunningham, Herie, Martin & Turner, 1998).

As an adjunct to, or even template for, Twelve-Step programs, *"institutional therapeutic community"* (ITC) programs have been at least provisionally implemented in some correctional institutions and represent the prevalent model for *residential substance abuse treatment* (R-SAT) programs in the community, especially those in which correctional or court-referred clients represent the majority (Mrad & Krasnoff, 1976; Knight, Simpson, Chatham & Camacho, 1997; McCorkel, Harrison & Inciardi, 1998; Siege, Wang, Carlson, Falck, Rahman & Fine, 1999; Knight, Hiller, Broome & D. W. Simpson, 2000). With appropriate modifications, correctional ITC programs apply principles evolved from the introduction of "milieu therapy" in psychiatric institutions in the 1920s (Rosenbaum, 1976).

Application of the pivotal premise that a patient's entire institutional experience, and not merely the hour or two that he/she spends with a psychiatrist each week, should yield therapeutic benefit literally revolutionized the operation of psychiatric hospitals, so that a variety of functions and services, ranging from physical activities to occupational therapy and group therapy, were introduced. Because patients and staff, including nurses and ward orderlies, began to interact intensely with each other in a variety of social configurations, a sense of community typically ensued, in which each member sought to contribute to the well-being of other members.

In correctional institutions, contemporary ITC units have tended to focus on drug offenders. Despite inherent hierarchical and prospectively adversarial relationships, corrections officers as well as rehabilitation personnel are regarded as full members of correctional ITCs. Perhaps for that reason, membership in such units is typically limited to offenders who have had few prior convictions and have incurred few disciplinary infractions during the present confinement. It is normatively (and by design) the case that group discussion, whether leaderless or peer-led, comes to occupy a major portion of time that is not otherwise consumed with institutional routines.

Family intervention services are sometimes incorporated into the template, especially in programs targeted at juvenile offenders. These services range from customary family counseling (Stringfield, 1977) and psychodidactic modalities (Sagatun, 1991; Bayse, Allgood & Van Wyk, 1992) to more aggressive and intensive "family empowerment programs" (Cameron & Cadell, 1999; Dembo, Ramirez-Garnica, Rollie & Schmeidler, 2000; Dembo, Ramirez-Garnica, Rollie, Schmeidler, Livingston & Hartsfield, 2000) aimed at family preservation combined with parent education and reduction of recidivism. It is not infrequent that parents themselves require access to a variety of social, educational, or mental health services.

Once a staple in the armamentarium of behavior therapy, *token economy programs* (Ottomanelli, 1976, 2001; Toch, 1988) that "reward" participants for positive behavior and "fine" them for negative behavior are often incorporated into both ITC and R-SAT modalities. In what is likely the most ambitious token economy ever implemented (Ault & Weston, 1975), inmates confined in the prisons of Georgia were permitted to "earn" release on parole by accumulating the requisite number of tokens.

THE PROBLEM OF COERCED TREATMENT

Although society may believe that it is more appropriate to treat than to punish drug abusers (that is to say, that drug abusers "need" treatment), there is scant evidence that the abusers themselves generally "want" treatment. Indeed, there is reason to believe that criminally-offending drug abusers frequently prove resistant to rehabilitation services of virtually every sort, for a variety of reasons ranging from the ego-syntonic character both of the abuse of drugs itself (surely self-rewarding) and of certain disorders prevalent in correctional populations (e.g., mania, psychopathic deviation) to a fixed perception that whatever is offered under the benefice of the correctional authority will ultimately prove punitive. For such reasons, offenders are likely to perceive as *coercive and to be resisted* (Sagatun, 1981; Polchin, 1999; Knight, Hiller, Broome & Simpson, 2000; Shearer, 2000) even the most non-intrusive, non-invasive modalities of treatment for what they do *not* perceive as disorders.

It is not necessary to underscore that the clinical skills required when prospective clients believe themselves to be coerced into treatment may differ substantially from those required when clients are eager for treatment for disorders, problems, or issues they have identified themselves. Operationally, it is not self-evident that evolving disorder-specific "standards of care" and statements of "empirically validated treatments" derived from clinical work with the "civilian" population apply with equal cogency to correctional clients coerced into treatment.

SUMMARY

Although its remote origins can be traced to the end of prohibition with the repeal of the Volstead Act in 1933, the nation's "war on drugs" gathered massive strength in the early days of the Reagan administration. During the 1980s and 1990s, the decision of the nation, expressed through its legislators, seemed to be to "criminalize" drug use or abuse through imposition of harsh penalties for what had earlier been statutorily defined as relatively minor offenses and by eliminating judicial discretion in sentencing, so that mandatory incarceration was required for many offenses. Yet by 2000, the voters of California, the Governor and criminal court judges of New York, and even the nation's "drug czar" had decided that they would rather, as described by the *New York Times*, "treat then fight." This paper has situated that sea change in posture within a context of oscillation toward the goals of corrections generally during an era in which "therapeutic nihilism" and "just deserts" appeared to have carried the day.

REFERENCES

Allen, F.A. 1981. *The Decline of the Rehabilitative Ideal: Penal Policy and Social Purpose*. New Haven: Yale University Press.

American Friends Service Committee. 1971. *Struggle for Justice*. New York: Hill & Wang.

Anderson, D.B. 1999. Problem gambling among incarcerated male felons. *Journal of Offender Rehabilitation, 28 (3/4)*, 113-128.

Ault, A.C., & P.L. Weston. 1975. *Project PERM–Permanent Earned Release Model.* Atlanta: Georgia State Department of Corrections & Offender Rehabilitation, 1975.

Badger, D., P. Vaughn, M. Woodward & P. Williams. 1999. Planning to meet the needs of offenders with mental disorders in the United States. *Psychiatric Services, 50 (12),* 1624-1627.

Baum, D. 1991. *Smoke and Mirrors: The War on Drugs and the Politics of Failure.* Boston: Little, Brown.

Bayse, D.J., S.M. Allgood & P.C. Van Wyk. 1992. Locus of control, narcissism, and family life education in correctional rehabilitation. *Journal of Offender Rehabilitation, 17 (3/4),* 47-64.

Beck, A.J. 2000. *Bureau of Justice Statistics Bulletin: Prisoners in 1999.* Washington: Office of Justice Programs, US Department of Justice. Bulletin NCJ 183476.

Bowman, G., S. Hakim & P. Seidenstat (Eds.). 1993. *Privatizing Correctional Institutions.* New Brunswick, NJ: Transaction Publishers.

Cameron, G., & S. Cadell. 1999. Fostering empowering participation in prevention programs for disadvantaged children and families: Lessons from ten demonstrations sites. *Canadian Journal of Community Mental Health, 18 (1),* 105-122.

Clement, M. 1997-a. *Juvenile Justice System: Law and Process.* Newton, MA: Butterworth-Heinemann.

Clement, M. 1997-b. New treatment for drug-abusing women offenders in Virginia. *Journal of Offender Rehabilitation, 25 (1/2),* 61-82.

Cotte, J. 1997. Chances, trances, and lots of slots: Gambling motives and consumption experiences. *Journal of Leisure Research, 29 (4),* 380-406.

Cullen, F.T., & K.E. Gilbert. 1982. *Reaffirming Rehabilitation.* Cincinnati: Anderson.

Cunningham, J.A., M. Herie, G. Martin & B.J. Turner. 1998. Training probation and parole officers to provide substance abuse treatment: A field test. *Journal of Offender Rehabilitation, 27 (1/2),* 167-178.

Daniel, C., & C. Dodd. 1990. Covert sensitization treatment in the elimination of alcohol-related crime in incarcerated young offenders. *Journal of Offender Rehabilitation, 16 (1/2),* 123-137.

Dembo, R., G. Ramirez-Garnica, M.W. Rollie & J. Schmeidler. 2000. Impact of a family empowerment intervention on youth recidivism. *Journal of Offender Rehabilitation, 30 (3/4),* 59-98.

Dembo, R., G. Ramirez-Garnica, M.W. Rollie, J. Schmeidler, S. Livingston & A. Hartsfield. 2000. Youth recidivism twelve months after a family empowerment intervention: Final report. *Journal of Offender Rehabilitation, 31 (3/4),* 29-66.

Demone, H.W., & M. Gibelman. 1990. "Privatizing" the treatment of criminal offenders. *Journal of Offender Counseling, Services & Rehabilitation, 15 (1),* 7-26.

Feinberg, S., & P. Gramsbach. 1979. An assessment of the accuracy of "The Effectiveness of Correctional Treatment." In L. Sechrest, S. O. White & E.D. Brown (Eds.), *The Rehabilitation of Criminal Offenders: Problems and Prospects.* Washington: National Academy of Sciences. Pp. 119-147.

Feld, B.C. 1998. Juvenile and criminal justice systems' responses to youth violence. In M. Tonry & H. Moore (Eds.), *Youth Violence.* Chicago: University of Chicago Press.

Fingarette, H. 1988. *Heavy Drinking: The Myth of Alcoholism as a Disease.* Berkeley, CA: University of California Press.

Fingarette, H. 1990. We should reject the disease concept of alcoholism. *Harvard Medical School Mental Health Letter, 6 (8)*, 4-6.

Foucault, M. 1978. *Discipline and Punish: The Birth of the Prison.* New York: Pantheon.

Fowler, R.D. 1976. Sweeping reforms ordered in Alabama prisons. *APA Monitor, 7 (4)*, 1, 15.

Fowler, R.D. 1988. Assessment for decision in a correctional setting. In D.R. Peterson & D.B. Fishman (Eds.), *Assessment for Decision.* New Brunswick, NJ: Rutgers University Press.

Gendreau, P., & B. Ross. 1979. Effective correctional treatment: Bibliotherapy for cynics. *Crime & Delinquency, 25 (4)*, 463-489.

Gendreau, P., & D.A. Andrews. 1990. Tertiary prevention: What the meta-analyses of the offender treatment literature tell us about "what works." *Canadian Journal of Criminology, 32 (1)*, 173-184.

Glaser, D. 1979. Achieving better questions: A half century's progress in correctional research. *Federal Probation, 39 (3)*, 3-9.

Glatt, M.M. 1974. *Drugs, Society, and Man: A Guide to Addiction and Its Treatment.* New York: John Wiley & Sons.

Golann, S., & W.J. Fremouw. 1976. *The Right to Treatment for Mental Patients.* New York: Irvington.

Gormally, J.G., S.L. Brodsky, C.B. Clements & R. Fowler. 1972. *Minimum Mental Health Standards for the Alabama Correctional System.* University, AL: Center for Correctional Psychology, University of Alabama.

Greer, C., A. Lawson, S. Baldwin & S. Cochrane. 1990. Alcohol abuse and the young offender: Alcohol education as an alternative to custodial sentencing. *Journal of Offender Counseling, Services & Rehabilitation, 15 (1)*, 131-145.

Hennessy, J.J. 2001. Drug courts in operation. *Journal of Offender Rehabilitation, 33 (4)*, 1-10.

Hirschel, J.D., & J.R. Keny. 1990. Outpatient treatment for substance-abusing offenders. *Journal of Offender Counseling, Services & Rehabilitation, 15 (1)*, 111-130.

Hofmann, Frederick G., & Adele D. Hofmann. 1975. *A Handbook on Drug and Alcohol Abuse: The Biomedical Aspects.* New York: Oxford University Press.

Hollin, C.R. 1990. *Cognitive-Behavioral Interventions with Young Offenders.* New York: Pergamon.

Hollin, C.R. 1999. Treatment programs for offenders: Meta-analysis, "what works," and beyond. *International Journal of Law & Psychiatry, 22 (3/4)*, 361-372.

Jenkins, L.A. 1995. Pre-trial diversion strategies for drug involved offenders: Focus on social work involvement. *Journal of Offender Rehabilitation, 22 (3/4)*, 129-140.

Karper, L.P., A.L. Bennett, J.J. Erdos & J.H. Krystal. 1994. Antipsychotics, lithium, benzodiazepines, beta-blockers. In M. Hillbrand & N.J. Pallone (Eds.), *The Psychobiology of Aggression: Engines, Measurement, Control.* New York: Haworth Press. Pp. 203-222.

Kempf-Leonard, K., & E.S.L. Peterson. 2000. Expanding realms of the new penology: The advent of actuarial justice for juveniles. *Punishment & Society, 2 (1)*, 66-97.

Knight, K., D.W. Simpson & D.F. Danserau. 1994. Knowledge mapping: A psychoeducational tool in drug abuse relapse prevention training. *Journal of Offender Rehabilitation, 20 (3/4)*, 187-206.

Knight, K., D.W. Simpson, L.R. Chatham & L.M. Camacho. 1997. An assessment of prison-based drug treatment: Texas' in-prison therapeutic community program. *Journal of Offender Rehabilitation, 24 (3/4)*, 75-100.

Knight, K., M.L. Hiller, K.M. Broome & D.W. Simpson. 2000. Legal pressure, treatment readiness and engagement in long-term residential programs. *Journal of Offender Rehabilitation, 31 (1/2)*, 101-116.

Kronick, R.F. 1993. Private vs. public care for juvenile offenders. *Journal of Offender Rehabilitation, 19 (3/4)*, 191-104.

Lindner, R.M. 1949. *Handbook of Correctional Psychology.* New York: Philosophical Library.

Lipton, D. 1994. The correctional opportunity: Pathways to drug treatment for offenders. *Journal of Drug Issues, 24 (4)*, 331-348.

Lipton, D. 1995. CDATE: Updating *The Effectiveness of Correctional Treatment* 25 years later. *Journal of Offender Rehabilitation, 22 (1/2)*, 1-20.

Lipton, D. 1998. Treatment for drug abusing offenders during correctional supervision: A nationwide overview. *Journal of Offender Rehabilitation, 26 (3/4)*, 1-46.

Lipton, D., R. Martinson & J. Wilks. 1975. *The Effectiveness of Correctional Treatment: A Survey of Treatment Evaluation Studies.* New York: Praeger.

Loesel, F. 1993. The effectiveness of treatment in institutional and community settings. *Criminal Behaviour & Mental Health, 3 (4)*, 416-437.

Loesel, F. 1995. Increasing the consensus in the evaluation of offender rehabilitation: Lessons from recent research syntheses. *Psychology, Crime & Law, 2 (1)*, 19-39.

Lucker, G.W., & J.R. Osti. 1997. Reduced recidivism among first-time DWI offenders as a correlate of pre-trial intervention. *Journal of Offender Rehabilitation, 24 (3/4)*, 1-18.

Maguire, K., & A.L. Pastore (Eds.). 1999. *Sourcebook of Criminal Justice Statistics.* Washington: Bureau of Justice Statistics, US Department of Justice.

Martinson, R. 1974. What works?–Questions and answers about prison reform. *Public Interest, 35 (1)*, 22-54.

Martinson, R. 1976. California research at the crossroads. *Crime & Delinquency, 12 (2)*, 189-199.

Matthews, W.G. 1980. Pretrial diversion screening: An analysis of differential labeling categories on sentencing outcomes. *Journal of Offender Counseling, Services & Rehabilitation, 4 (4)*, 369-380.

Mayer, C. 1990. *Survey of Case Law Establishing Constitutional Minima for the Provision of Mental Health Services to Psychiatrically Involved Inmates.* Albany, NY: Albany Law School.

McCorkel, J., L.D. Harrison & J. Inciardi. 1998. How treatment is constructed among graduates and dropout in a prison therapeutic community for women. *Journal of Offender Rehabilitation, 27 (3/4)*, 37-60.

McGaha, J.E. 1993. Alcoholism and the chemically dependent family: A study of adult felons on probation. *Journal of Offender Rehabilitation, 19 (3/4)*, 57-70.

Morris, N. 1974. *The Future of Imprisonment.* Chicago: University of Chicago Press.

Mrad, D.F., & A.G. Krasnoff. 1976. Use of the MMPI and demographic variables in predicting dropouts from a correctional therapeutic community. *Offender Rehabilitation, 1 (2)*, 193-202.

Nadelmann, E.A. 1993. *Cops Across Borders: The Internationalization of U.S. Criminal Law Enforcement*. University Park, PA: Pennsylvania State University Press.

Newbern, D., D.F. Danserau & S.M. Dees. 1997. Node-link mapping in substance abuse: Probationers' ratings of group counseling. *Journal of Offender Rehabilitation, 25 (1/2)*, 83-96.

Ottomanelli, G. 1976. Follow-up of a token economy applied to civilly-committed heroin addicts. *International Journal of the Addictions*, 1976, *11 (10)*, 793-806.

Ottomanelli, G. 2001. *Assessment and Treatment of Chemical Dependency*. Westport, CT: Praeger.

Pallone, N.J. 1991. *Mental Disorder among Prisoners: Toward an Epidemiologic Inventory*. New Brunswick, NJ: Transaction Publishers.

Pallone, N.J., & J.J. Hennessy. 1996. *Tinder-Box Criminal Aggression: Neuropsychology, Demography, Phenomenology*. New Brunswick, NJ: Transaction Publishers.

Pallone, N.J., & D.S. LaRosa. 1979. Mental health specialists and services in correctional facilities: Who does what? *Offender Rehabilitation, 4 (1)*, 33-41.

Pallone, N.J., J.J. Hennessy & D.S. LaRosa. 1980. Professional psychology in state correctional institutions: Present status and alternate futures. *Professional Psychology, 11 (5)*, 755-763.

Penrose, L.S. 1939. Mental disease and crime: Outline of a comparative study of European statistics. *Medical Psychology, 19 (1)*, 1-15.

Perez-Pena, R. 2001. Pataki presents his plan to ease state drug laws. *New York Times*, January 18, A-9.

Peters, R.H., & H.A. Hills. 1999. Community treatment and supervision strategies for offenders with co-occurring disorders: What works. In E. Latessa (Ed.), *Strategic Solutions: The International Community Corrections Association Examines Substance Abuse*. Lanham, MD: American Correctional Association.

Peters, R.H., & M.R. Murrin. 2000. Effectiveness of treatment-based drug courts in reducing criminal recidivism. *Criminal Justice & Behavior, 27 (1)*, 72-96.

Peters, R.H., R.L. May & W.D. Kearns. 1992. Drug treatment in jails: Results of a nationwide survey. *Journal of Criminal Justice, 20 (4)*, 283-295.

Peters, R.H., W.D. Kearns, M.R. Murrin, A.S. Dolente & R.L. May. 1993. Examining the effectiveness of in-jail substance abuse treatment. *Journal of Offender Rehabilitation, 19 (3/4)*, 1-40.

Peters, R.H., P.E. Greenbaum, J.F. Edens, C.R. Carter & M.M. Ortiz. 1998. Prevalence of DSM-IV substance abuse and dependence disorders among prison inmates. *American Journal of Drug & Alcohol Abuse, 24 (4)*, 573-587.

Polchin, D.L. 1999. Criminal justice coercion in the treatment of alcohol problems: An examination of subgroups. *Journal of Psychoactive Drugs, 31 (2)*, 137-143.

RAND Corporation, Office of External Communications. 2002. RAND study casts doubt on claims that marijuana acts as "gateway" to use of cocaine and heroin. Santa Monica, CA: The Corporation, December 2 (Available at oec@rand.org.).

Redondo, S., J. Sanchez-Meca & V. Garrido. 1999. The influence of treatment programmes on the recidivism of juvenile and adult offenders: An European meta-analytic review. *Psychology, Crime & Law, 5 (3)* 251-278.

Ronel, N. 1998. Narcotics Anonymous: Understanding "the bridge of recovery." *Journal of Offender Rehabilitation, 27 (1/2)*, 179-198.

Rose, S.R. 1997. Analysis of a juvenile court diversion program. *Journal of Offender Rehabilitation, 24 (3/4)*, 153-162.

Rosenbaum, M. 1976. Group psychotherapies. In B.B. Wolman (Ed.), *Therapist's Handbook: Treatment Methods for Mental Disorders.* New York: Van Nostrand Reinhold. Pp. 163-183.

Sagatun, I.J. 1981. The effects of court-ordered therapy on incest offenders. *Journal of Offender Counseling, Services & Rehabilitation, 5, (3/4)*, 99-104.

Sagatun, I.J. 1991. Attributions of delinquency by delinquent minors, their families, and probation officers. *Journal of Offender Rehabilitation, 16 (3/4)*, 43-59.

Scarpitti, F.R., J.A. Inciardi & A.E. Pottieger. 1993. Process evaluation techniques for corrections-based drug treatment programs. *Journal of Offender Rehabilitation, 19 (3/4)*, 71-80.

Schnapp, W.B., & R. Cannedy. 1998. Offenders with mental illness: Mental health and criminal justice best practices. *Administrative Policy & Mental Health, 25 (4)*, 463-466.

Scott, R.E.F., R.D. Hawkins & M. Farnsworth. 1994. Operation kick-it: Texas prisoners rehabilitate themselves by dissuading others. *Journal of Offender Rehabilitation, 20 (3/4)*, 207-215.

Sechrest, L., S. O. White & E.D. Brown (Eds.). 1979. *The Rehabilitation of Criminal Offenders: Problems and Prospects.* Washington: National Academy of Sciences.

Shamsie, J. 1981. Anti-social adolescents: Our treatments are not working–Where do we go from here? *Annual Progress in Child Psychiatry & Child Development, 24 (2)*, 631-647.

Shearer, R.A. 2000. Coerced substance abuse counseling revisited. *Journal of Offender Rehabilitation, 30 (3/4)*, 153-171.

Sherman, M., & G. Hawkins. 1981. *Imprisonment in American: Choosing the Future.* Chicago: University of Chicago Press.

Siege, H.A., J. Wang, R.G. Carlson, R.S. Falck, A.M. Rahman & R.L. Fine. 1999. Ohio's prison-based therapeutic community treatment programs for substance abusers. *Journal of Offender Rehabilitation, 28 (3/4)*, 33-48.

Smith, M.L., G.V. Glass & T.I. Miller. 1980. *The Benefits of Psychotherapy.* Baltimore: Johns-Hopkins University Press.

Stringfield, N. 1977. The impact of family counseling in resocializing adolescent offenders within a positive peer treatment milieu. *Offender Rehabilitation, 1 (4)*, 349-360.

Substance Abuse and Mental Health Services Administration, Office of Applied Studies. *National Survey of Substance Abuse Treatment Services (N-SSATS): 2000. Data on Substance Abuse Treatment Facilities*, DASIS Series: S-16, DHHS Publication No. (SMA) 02-3668, Rockville, MD, 2002.

Szasz, T. 1992. *Our Right to Drugs: The Case for a Free Market.* New York: Praeger.

Taylor, W.B., & M.C. Brasswell. 1979. Reflections on penology: Retribution revisited. *Journal of Offender Counseling, Services & Rehabilitation, 4 (2)*, 109-120.

Tims, F., J. Inciardi, B. Fletcher & A. Horton. 1997. *The Effectiveness of Innovative Approaches in the Treatment of Drug Abuse.* Westport, CT: Greenwood.

Toch, H. 1988. Rewarding convicted offenders. *Federal Probation, 52 (2)*, 42-48.

von Hirsch, A. 1976. *Doing Justice: The Choice of Punishments.* New York: Hill & Wang.

von Hirsch, A. 1984. The ethics of selective incapacitation: Observations on the contemporary debate. *Crime & Delinquency, 30 (2)*, 175-194.

von Hirsch, A. 1985. *Past or Future Crimes: Deservedness and Dangerousness in the Sentencing of Criminals.* New Brunswick, NJ: Rutgers University Press.

von Hirsch, A. 1988. *Federal Sentencing Guidelines: The United States and Canadian Schemes Compared.* New York: Center for Research in Crime & Justice, School of Law, New York University.

Wagoner, J.L., & N.J. Piazza. 1993. Group therapy for adult substance abusers on probation. *Journal of Offender Rehabilitation, 19 (3/4)*, 41-56.

Welch. M. 1999. *Punishment in America: Social Control and the Ironies of Imprisonment.* Beverly Hills: Sage.

Wexler, H.K., J. Blackmore & D. Lipton. 1991. Project REFORM: Developing a drug abuse treatment strategy for corrections. *Journal of Drug Issues, 21 (2)*, 469-490.

Wildman, R.W. 2000. General theory of addictions provides solid guidance for treatment of problem gamblers. *Report on Problem Gambling, 1, 1*, 1, 2, 12.

Wren, Christopher S. 2001. A drug warrior who would rather treat than fight. *New York Times*, January 8, B-9.

Zimring, F.E. 1998. Toward a jurisprudence of youth violence. In M. Tonry & M.H. Moore (Eds.), *Youth Violence.* Chicago: University of Chicago Press. Pp. 477-501.

AUTHORS' NOTES

Nathaniel J. Pallone, PhD, is University Distinguished Professor (Psychology), Center of Alcohol Studies, at Rutgers–The State University of New Jersey, where he previously served as dean and as academic vice president. Early in his career, he served for six years as senior consulting psychologist to the New York State Narcotics Addiction Control Commission.

James J. Hennessy, PhD, is a professor and former chairperson, Division of Psychological and Educational Services, Graduate School of Education, Fordham University, New York City. Among his current research activities, he serves as the independent evaluation consultant to drug courts in the cities of Yonkers and Mount Vernon in Westchester County, New York.

Their joint books include *Drug Courts in Operation: Current Research* (Haworth, 2001); *Tinder-Box Criminal Aggression: Neuropsychology, Demography, Phenomenology* (Transaction, 1996); *Fraud and Fallible Judgment: Varieties of Deception in the Social and Behavioral Sciences* (Transaction, 1995); and *Criminal Behavior: A Process Psychology Analysis* (Transaction, 1992).

Address correspondence to Dr. N. J. Pallone, 215 Smithers Hall, Center of Alcohol Studies, Rutgers–The State University, New Brunswick, NJ 08901 (E-mail: NJP1800@ aol.com).

Treating Substance Abusers in Correctional Contexts: New Understandings, New Modalities. Pp. 27-46.
10.1300/J076v37n03_02

Perceptions of a Prison-Based Substance Abuse Treatment Program Among Some Staff and Participants

SARAH GOODRUM

Department of Anthropology and Sociology, Centre College

MICHELE STATON

University of Kentucky Center on Drug and Alcohol Research

CARL LEUKEFELD

Department of Behavioral Science, University of Kentucky

J. MATTHEW WEBSTER

University of Kentucky Center on Drug and Alcohol Research

RICHARD T. PURVIS

Kentucky Department of Corrections

ABSTRACT Almost 90% of all State and Federal prisons in the U.S. offer some form of substance abuse counseling, and one in eight prisoners have participated in a substance abuse treatment program while incarcerated. Evidence indicates that these programs can be successful in stopping prisoners' substance abuse. While some data are available about the success of these programs, little is known about program administrators', counselors' and participants' experiences with and perceptions of these treatment programs. These experiences and perceptions remain important because they may be helpful for understanding areas of agreement and conflict in staff-participant relationships. The more understanding we have for these relationships, the more likely it is that we will be able to improve staff-participant communications, program effectiveness, and participant success. The results suggest similarities and differences between staff and participants in the areas of participant motivation, staff-participant communication, race, institutional support, and counselor contacts. Implications of the results of this inquiry for prison-based substance abuse treatment programs are discussed. *[Article copies available for a fee from The Haworth Document Delivery Service: 1-800-HAWORTH. E-mail address: <docdelivery@haworthpress.com> Website: <http://www.HaworthPress.com> © 2003 by The Haworth Press, Inc. All rights reserved.]*

KEYWORDS Substance abuse treatment, prison, perceptions, qualitative

For more than 30 years, researchers, practitioners, and legislators have recognized the importance of drug treatment programs for incarcerated populations (Leukefeld, Tims, & Farabee, 2002; Martin, Butzin, Saum, & Inciardi, 1999) and for reducing offenders' rates of recidivism and substance relapse (see Griffith, Hiller, Knight, & Simpson, 1999). As of 1997, more than 80% of State prisoners reported having used drugs in their lifetime, 57% reported having used drugs in the month prior to their offense, and 33% reported having used drugs at the time of the offense (Mumola, 1999). Almost 90% of State and Federal prisons offer some type of drug and alcohol counseling (Stephan, 1997). One-third of State prisoners reported having participated in a substance abuse treatment program in their lifetimes, and one in eight prisoners reported having participated in a substance abuse program during incarceration (Mumola, 1999).

Some things are known about prison-based substance abuse treatment program successes (Inciardi, Surratt, Martin, & Hooper, 2002; Wexler, Melnick, Lowe, & Peters, 1999). For example, a supportive program environment, staff members' understanding of clients' needs, and clients' genuine interest in treatment improve client success (Joe, Simpson, & Broome, 1998; Yih-Ing, 1995). However, little is known about staff and clients' experiences with and perceptions of prison-based substance abuse treatment (for exceptions see McCollum & Trepper, 1995; McCorkel, Harrison, & Inciardi, 1998; Murdock, McCoy, McBride, & Weppner, 1980). These views remain critical for understanding the program and its outcomes. Knowing staff members' and participants' perceptions about what is helpful and not so helpful about the program will inform us about how to revise it. This study seeks to understand those views through an analysis of in-depth interviews with administrators, counselors, and participants involved in a prison-based substance abuse treatment program in Kentucky. The goals of this research are to: (1) identify staff members' perceptions of the program and its participants, (2) identify participants' experiences with and perceptions of the program and its staff, and (3) examine the areas of conflict and agreement in participant and staff perceptions. The presentation of the findings is organized around the main themes in the data, and for each theme, we delineate the areas of agreement and disagreement in staff members' and participants' perceptions and experiences.

LITERATURE REVIEW

Staff Members

The substance abuse literature indicates that there is a need for prison-based substance abuse treatment. Lo and Stevens (2000) find that approximately one-third of incoming prisoners had used at least three substances. In substance abuse treatment programs, administrators and counselors play a pivotal role in the rehabilitation of drug-abusing offenders, and there is some evidence to suggest that these staff members' perceptions of the program and its participants also influence program outcomes. Finn (1994, p. 326) reports, "[S]taff found that their failure to understand these clients' cultural values was in large measure responsible for the high discharge rate." A staff person who is unable to take the perspective (or role) of the other (i.e., put him or herself in the client's shoes) may not be able to adequately meet the needs of the client. According to symbolic interactionist theory, taking the role of the other involves imagining how another person may feel about or react to a situation; role-taking allows the individual to plan his or her behavior in anticipation of another's feeling or reaction (Mead, 1934). In addition, research and theory in symbolic interactionism suggest that a person's ability to take the role of the other, in this case, the participant, can smooth subsequent interactions (Mead, 1934).

The notion of role-taking has implications for staff members' interactions with participants from other racial groups or cultures (e.g., rural or urban community) in substance abuse treatment. "[M]any programs already appear to have difficulty recruiting, retaining, and successfully treating minority clients" (Finn, 1994, pp. 325). However, therapists with strong counseling abilities can facilitate increased client success, and therapists that build supportive relationships with clients are very effective (Yih-Ing, 1995). Yih-Ing (1995) recognizes that the increased agreement between staff members and clients, particularly in the areas of client issues, treatment needs, and treatment goals, can bring increased client success.

There is some evidence to suggest, however, that problems arise when the staff member's ability to execute his or her plan for treatment is compromised by larger program problems, such as program support. "[I]mproved counselor efficacy cannot be achieved without the appropriate supportive program environment" (Yih-Ing, 1995, pp. 2-3). To address this problem, Broome, Knight, Hiller, and Simpson (1996) argue that research on substance abuse treatment should examine the contexts underlying treatment programs to better understand program experience and success, and the authors recommend that future research consider the role of perceptions in treatment. "[T]he best way to begin understanding the various interactions (Cronbach, 1982a, 1982b) between the client, the counselor, and the program is to obtain the richest possible description of its context and process" (Yih-Ing, 1995, p. 4). In-depth interviewing provides detailed information about these contexts, and this type of data offers rich insight into staff members' and participants' experiences.

Participants

The substance abuse literature also indicates that participant motivation, means of referral, perceptions, and program context play a role in participant success following treatment. Joe, Simpson, and Broome (1998) find that clients' motivation for drug abuse treatment prior to entering treatment affects their engagement and retention. Client motivation influenced the quality of the therapeutic relationship (Simpson, Joe, Rowan-Szal, & Greener, 1997), and it also improved clients' views of counselor competence (Broome et al., 1996). This study examined staff members' and participants' views of motivation for treatment, as well as the way those views differed by perspectives (e.g., staff or participant). While motivation plays an important role in participants' success, the means of their referral does not appear to be as instrumental. DeLeon (1988) finds no evidence to support the idea that the legal or non-legal referral status influenced client success. Legally referred clients, however, remained in treatment longer than non-legally referred clients, which can positively affect success (DeLeon, 1988). In addition, clients appear to hold more confidence in rehabilitated counselors (Winick, 1990-91). The clients' perception that a counselor can truly relate to their situation appears to be important to clients, and it may also influence their interest in and ability to discontinue their drug use following treatment. These rehabilitated counselors may give participants the hope that if he or she can do it, I can also. Clients in a prison-based substance abuse treatment program who had positive views of counselors' competence were 39% less likely to be re-arrested, suggesting that clients' perceptions of counselors can affect client success (Broome et al., 1996). This study examined participants' views of the program and its staff to better understand the meaning of competence.

DATA AND METHODS

This study emerges from a larger project on drug treatment and health services utilization. The data come from in-depth interviews with 2 administrators, 5 counselors, and 18 participants, which were conducted over a 4-year period from 1998 to 2001 (for additional information, see Staton, Leukefeld,

Logan, & Purvis, 2000). The program had one administrator, who was interviewed each year. The administrator changed in the second year of the study, which explains the participation of two administrators over the course of the study. The program had approximately 6 counselors at any one time, and 2 counselors (or approximately 33% of the counselors on staff) were interviewed each year. The program had approximately 100 participants at any one time, and 4-6 participants were interviewed each year. Each interview transcript comprised approximately 2-3 pages of single-spaced type and a total of 60 pages of transcript data were used for this research.

The transcriptions were analyzed and coded by the lead author using Lofland and Lofland's (1995) techniques for qualitative data analysis, which are explained in more detail here. The analysis of the transcript data involved two readings: an "initial" and then a "focused" reading (Charmaz, 1983; Maynard, 1996). The goal during the initial reading was to make brief notes about the recurrent themes in interviewees' responses; these notes were used to develop and refine codes suggested in (1) previous research and (2) interviewees' responses. In previous research, "participant motivation" and "staff-participant communication" have emerged as important in understanding staff members' and participants' experiences in substance abuse treatment programs. Thus, in the course of the initial reading, the lead author reviewed the transcripts for the mention of these issues. Those issues appeared in interviewees' responses and were subsequently developed as codes, a common technique in qualitative data analysis (see also Maynard, 1996). Several codes were subsequently developed from interviewees' responses, including the issues of "institutional support" and "counselor contact."

The goal during the focused reading was to manually code the data. During the focused reading, each transcript was read ten times, once for each code (see Appendix for the ten codes and frequency of each in the data). The text illustrating each code was highlighted and labeled (or coded) in the left margin of the transcript. Once all of the transcripts were coded, the highlighted and coded text was copied into a separate Word document. When an interviewee's response was identified as illustrating a specific code, the response and the interviewee's identification number were copied into a file organized by codes. There were responses that illustrated more than one of the ten codes. When a response reflected more than one code, the response was copied under all relevant codes with a comment noting the cross-listed codes. For example, interviewees' comments about the underrepresentation of minorities on the program staff was coded under both "race" and "program challenges." In the end, the coded data file comprised 22 pages of single-spaced type.

It is important to note that some codes emerged infrequently in subjects' responses and others did not yield any variation in interviewees' responses. The data from these codes, including gender, participant change, staff-administration communication, and program positives, are not reported here. In the results section, we present the responses most clearly illustrating the theme embodied in the code, while noting exceptions to the general theme. To protect interviewees' confidentiality, we assigned numbers to each interviewee (e.g., Counselor 1, Counselor 2, Participant 1); we also note the year of the study in which the interview was conducted. The year notation allowed us to consider the possibility that the responses changed over time, and the evidence suggests that responses did change over time, becoming more positive in years 3 and 4 than in year 1. The program made gradual changes over the course of the 4-year study, and many of the changes parallel suggestions made by staff and participants in the interviews. However, whether those changes were a direct result of the data collected from the in-depth interviews or to the initiative of staff to incorporate change is unknown.

Program Profile

In 1992, the Kentucky Task Force on Substance Abuse Treatment recommended that Kentucky prisons offer substance abuse treatment, and in June 1992, the Kentucky State Reformatory started the Substance Abuse Program (SAP). The Reformatory is a medium security prison located in LaGrange and it houses 1,391 male prisoners. SAP participants can participate in individual and group counseling sessions, as well as education classes. The program started as 60 days and is now 180 days, and it uses 12-step programming and cognition and behavior training (see also Staton et al., 2000). One counselor described the goal of the program:

> [The overall treatment philosophy of SAP] is about people growing up and being responsible individuals by changing not only their addictions, but also their behavior. [Our ultimate] goal is to make society better by reducing the number of inmates. (Counselor 2, Year 1)

RESULTS

Several themes emerged in the data (across all 3 types of interviewees), including the issues of participant motivation, staff-participant communication, race, institutional support, and counselor contacts. Staff members and participants appear to agree, for the most part, on the issues of participant motivation and staff-participant communication; however, interesting differences exist in staff members' and participants' views of the program's challenges, including racial diversities, institutional support, and counselor contacts. The findings are presented in two sections: similarities in perceptions and differences in perceptions. Within these two sections, staff members' and participants' perceptions on the issues are compared and contrasted in an attempt to explain the role these perceptions play in treatment and outcomes. Changes in the nature of the themes occurring over the course of the 4-year study are also noted.

Similarities in Perceptions

Participant Motivation

Staff members and participants agreed that most participants' primary motivation for participating in this prison-based substance abuse program was for the parole opportunity it provided. Six of the seven staff members interviewed for the study reported parole as the biggest motivator for enrollment, and some staff questioned the genuineness of participants' help-seeking behavior. One explained:

> [Inmates join the program] almost exclusively because of the parole opportunity. Some [of the participants] say that they are there because the program will help them, but I feel that they may be insincere. (Counselor 1, Year 1)

The parole opportunity presents a dilemma for prison and program staff. An administrator recognized that although the program was "voluntary," many inmates felt obligated to enroll in it when the parole board recommended it to them in their parole board hearings. He explained:

> Nothing is truly "volunteer" in prison. Most [inmates] are referred by the parole board [so it's a] systemic motivation.

He acknowledged the presence of both treatment and non-treatment oriented reasons for participants' involvement in the program. He said:

> The reason participants want to participate include appeasing the parole board, realizing the problems that drugs and alcohol have caused in their lives, and having a desire to make changes in their lives. Others may apply for the program because they know that [the Kentucky State Reformatory] is a pretty easy place to do time. (Administrator 1, Year 1)

Participants agreed with staff members' perceptions of participant motivation. Fifty percent of participants agreed that they and other participants enrolled in the program for the parole opportunity. Two participants said:

> Honestly, [I wanted to participate in SAP] because of parole. I had recently been through a drug treatment program, and I am not sure that I really needed another program. (Participant 8, Year 1)

> [I wanted to participate in SAP because there was a] 90% chance you'd go home. (Participant 3, Year 1)

Some participants' responses suggest that this obligatory participation, however, diminished the quality of the experience for other more genuinely motivated participants in the program. Two participants believed:

> They should have a better way of getting rid of the people that don't want to learn from either the group or SAP all together. (Participant 4, Year 1)

> There are too many unmotivated or insincere people in the program. . . . They need a new way to evaluate people in the program. Kick those out that do not belong or do not want to be there for the right reasons. (Participant 5, Year 1)

The unmotivated participants particularly presented a problem for other group members in the small group meetings. These meetings were held regularly, and in them, participants met as a group of six to eight people with the supervision of a staff member to talk about their substance abuse problems. To encourage openness in these meetings, counselors instructed participants not to talk about the feelings and experiences shared by others outside of the group. This practice assured participants of their privacy and also provided participants with an opportunity to develop trust. The practice appeared to be very effective. Both staff and participants viewed the small group meetings as very enriching learning experiences, particularly for participants. One participant described:

> [The part of SAP I like the best is the] small group, because you're able to speak your mind, get feedback from the other guys, and they understand. (Participant 3, Year 1)

Another participant explained:

> [In the] small group, there is a close bond, feelings for each other, and [we] work with each other. (Participant 9, Year 3)

The unmotivated participant can, however, disrupt the dynamics of the small group meeting, and the productivity of these meetings and the quality of the participants' substance abuse treatment can be jeopardized when not all participants participate.

This issue presents a difficult dilemma for parole boards, prison staff, and program staff in prison-based treatment programs (e.g., violence prevention, G.E.D.) around the U.S. Some evidence suggests that while participants may not enroll in the program voluntarily, they often grow to appreciate and accept the treatment program in time. One participant admitted:

I did not necessarily want to enter the program. I was "made" to, but now I know how much it will help me to get better and make parole. (Participant 6, Year 1)

Thus, prison-based treatment program staff members recognize and accept the value of systemic motivation in the long term. This type of motivation can ensure that program enrollment figures remain consistent. The question becomes: how can prison staff encourage self-improvement and treatment without bringing insincere interest?

The Staff-Participant Relationship

Staff and participants agreed that they sometimes experienced difficulty in communicating with each other, but despite these communication difficulties both groups described the overall staff-participant relationship as a positive one. Here, staff members' and participants' perceptions of the staff-participant relationship is examined. When asked how they would describe the staff-participant relationship, six of the seven staff stated the relationship with participants was good considering the environment and the population. In describing the relationship, three counselors said:

Things are as smooth as can be; this is a tough environment. (Counselor 5, Year 4)

For the most part, it is respectful. Staff and inmates both have things that need to be accomplished. . . . Some conflict does occur, but these are infrequent. (Counselor 1, Year 1)

Overall, [the staff-participant relationship is] really good. There are problems; nothing's perfect. Considering this population, it's a good relationship overall. (Counselor 2, Year 1)

This counselor recognized that sometimes relationship difficulties emerged when:

[S]taff members placed themselves above the inmates with their educational knowledge. (Counselor 2, Year 1)

Part of the staff-participant relationship challenge arose from staff members' competing (and sometimes conflicting) responsibilities. One counselor elaborated:

[There is a] balancing act between treatment and corrections. Explaining this to the participant is difficult, [and] reconciling the differences can be hard. (Counselor 4, Year 4)

Compton and Galaway (1994) recognize the dilemma that the duties of authority and service bring, and the authors warned that authority can impinge on the principle of self-determination (or the opportunity to make decisions about the self). Staff members' responses indicated that they value self-determination, and as a result, they allowed time for participants to self-determine their treatment following their systemically motivated enrollment in the program. This gave participants the opportunity to acknowledge and accept their problem with substance abuse and to invest themselves fully in the program. One counselor explained that the staff did not seek to engage participants in a struggle for power. Instead, "We have to give them time to change [themselves]" (Counselor 3, Year 3).

Participants also described the staff-participant relationship in positive terms, and participants frequently referred to counselors' attitudes, listening skills, and availability as the most important aspects of the staff-participant relationship. Fourteen of the 18 participants said that the staff-participant relationship was good.

> Yes, [the counselors are] really helpful. All of them care. They have this job for a reason. They can relate and know how to change lives for the better. They give everyone the knowledge and skills to do this. (Participant 13, Year 3)

> [We have] a good relationship with the counselors. They are very easy to talk to. (Participant 7, Year 1)

> Yes, [the staff are helpful]. The counselors can be helpful. You can go talk to them if you need to with stuff like family problems. . . . My counselor is very accessible and easy to talk to. (Participant 2, Year 1)

Only four participants described the staff-participant relationship as less than good, and they cited counselors' attitudes, listening skills, and availability as the factors contributing to the problem. One of these four participants explained:

> [The relationship between staff and participants is] poor. [It is] hard to communicate with one another. The staff looks at us as criminals. They don't believe the things we say; it [is] always the staff who's right. (Participant 3, Year 1)

It is important to note that three of these four participants' responses came from year 1 interviews and only one of these four participants' responses came from a year 4 interview, suggesting that participants' perceptions of the staff-participant relationship improved over the course of the 4-year study.

Differences in Perceptions

The staff identified race, a lack of support from the larger prison system, and understaffing as the main challenges facing the program. Most participants, on the other hand, indicated that the two difficulties facing the program included counselors' lack of understanding for participants and the limited opportunities for participants to receive one-on-one counseling.

Race

Staff members' greatest concerns about the program involved two race-related issues: the racial differences among staff and participants and the number of minorities on staff. First, five of the seven staff members indicated that racial differences, in some cases discrimination, presented some difficulties.

> [There are] some race problems [in the program]. . . . Differences have come up between staff and participants. (Counselor 2, Year 1)

For the most part, these program staff did not believe that the race differences negatively affected staff members' treatment work with participants, but they did see these challenges as negatively affecting participants' success in the program, as well as participants' interactions with other participants. One counselor explained:

> This does not seem to be that much of a problem for the counselors; however, it can lead to problems among inmates [with discrimination]. (Counselor 1, Year 1)

In awareness of the challenges race played in the program, the program administrator and counselors attempted to address the role of perceptions of race in treatment. One counselor explained:

> [Counselors] talk about prejudice [and] hatred as barriers to recovery. (Counselor 2, Year 1)

Not all staff members believed that racial differences existed in the program. One counselor believed that the presence of gangs, not racial differences, presented a challenge to program staff. She addressed this challenge in her work by making participants aware of the things they shared in common and de-emphasizing the things that made them different.

> Not a whole lot of attention is drawn to differences. Recently, there has been a lot of gang-related activity, and the staff is not sure how to handle

it. I simply try to make the [participants] realize that they are similar [to each other] in certain ways despite differences. (Counselor 1, Year 1)

In a surprising and important difference in staff and participants' perceptions, participants did *not* report racial differences as a program challenge. In fact, only 4 of the 18 program participants interviewed indicated that race presented any sort of challenge or difficulty in the program. It is not clear why this difference of opinion exists. It may be that participants simply have more experience with racial differences and thus do not recognize it as a noteworthy "problem." It may also be that administrators and counselors are more aware of and sensitive to the challenges that race difficulties present than participants.

Diversity was the second race issue to emerge in the data. Administrators and counselors identified the racial diversity and diversity training for the staff as one challenge facing the program. Several staff members believed that minority male participants experienced difficulty relating to white female counselors, and these counselors felt an African-American counselor would have alleviated some of these difficulties. By the second year of the study, a new administrator had taken over the program; this administrator described:

> Some [participants] want to talk specifically to a same gender or race staff member. Young African-American males tend to prefer black male counselors. (Administrator 2, Year 4)

In recognition of the lack of racial diversity in the program and the issues it presented in participants' experiences, the program recruited and hired an African-American counselor in the fourth year of the study. In year 4 of the study, one counselor said:

> The addition of an African-American male [counselor] has been a plus. They relate to him very well; he is a positive role model. (Counselor 5, Year 4)

Similarly, staff recognized the presence of the diversity challenge. The program administrator acknowledged that in the first year of the study there was no formal diversity training for program counselors. He explained:

> No formal training in cultural diversity or awareness currently exists [in the program]. As a staff, [the counselors] have made efforts to educate themselves. African-American participants often want to know why this difference exists. (Administrator 1, Year 1)

Program participants did not describe the lack of racial diversity among the staff as a problem as often as staff members did, which is the second important difference to arise in staff and participants' perceptions of the program. Only 4 of 18 participants mentioned the underrepresentation of minorities on the staff as a program weakness. In the first year of the study, a few participants simply described this underrepresentation as a source of missed opportunities for understanding in the staff-participant relationship. One participant explained:

> They really need an African-American counselor to deal with the multitude of issues that only a black would understand. (Participant 4, Year 1)

By the fourth year of the study, one of these participants indicated that although there was still an underrepresentation of African-Americans among program counselors, "All counselors [were] in touch culturally" (Participant 17, Year 4).

The reasons for the differences in perceptions of race among staff and participants remain unclear. It maybe that participants' race influences their perceptions of racial diversity.

Institutional and Staff Support

Several counselors indicated that both they and the program functioned without the complete support of the larger organization and the program operated without adequate staff, and they viewed these as the second and third greatest challenges facing the program after the race issue. The perception of lack of support perhaps relates to the inability to fully enforce program rules, particularly at night and weekends when program staff are not in the building, and a sense of not having the full cooperation of prison security.

> [There is a] general lack of support from security. Within the institution [larger prison in which SAP is housed], [there is a] lack of support. (Counselor 3, Year 3)

> [We] are rarely full-staffed; mainly because of the pay; good people won't do the work you have to do for the money. (Counselor 3, Year 3)

One participant agreed that the program needed more counselors to improve the quantity and quality of treatment received.

> [I would like] more on-on-one time with counselors. They are so busy that you have to make an appointment. SAP should hire more counselors and make groups and classes smaller. (Participant 1, Year 1)

Similarly, Yih-Ing (1995:3) has noted, "[A]dditional therapy could provide meaningful benefits to opiate addicts treated in a methadone maintenance program, particularly those with significant psychiatric symptoms in addition to addiction."

Dormitory, Counselors, and Program Meetings

No single theme emerged as dominant in participants' responses to questions about challenges facing the program. Instead, participants identified a few different areas for program improvement, including the dormitory living conditions, counselor professionalism, counselor understanding, and the Alcoholic Anonymous and Narcotics Anonymous meetings. This presents another area where program staff and participants' perceptions of and experiences with the program differed. Staff did not mention these four issues. First, participants wanted the dormitory to have a cleaner environment, improved maintenance, and better ventilation and temperature control. Three participants explained:

> [T]here are a lot of things wrong with the . . . building. There are areas that constantly flood, and multiple other run-down characteristics. I hate that there is no privacy for the bathrooms. (Participant 6, Year 1)

> The dorm is in bad shape. They have many water leaks. (Participant 8, Year 1)

> My room is okay. It is adequately sized, but I hate the ventilation. The air is recycled and full of smoke. . . . It is unfair that I breathe the unhealthy air. . . . The dorm also has extreme temperature problems. (Participant 5, Year 1)

Second, five participants indicated a wish for counselors to be either more professional in their demeanor or inspirational in their approach to treatment. Two participants reported:

> The counselors need to be more sincere and more professional. (Participant 6, Year 1)

> [The staff is helpful] to a certain extent, with certain problems . . . [but there needs to be] more professionalism from the counselors (changing their attitudes in the way they look at people) and making the program more interesting. (Participant 3, Year 1)

Third, while 8 of the 18 participants interviewed described counselors as helpful, good listeners, and accessible (for more details, see the section on the staff-participant relationship), 5 participants indicated that they thought the program's counselors could be more understanding. Two of these participants elaborated:

> The counselors need to be more understanding and more motivating. They are uninspiring most of the time. (Participant 4, Year 1)

Counselors should be more understanding on issues outside of class. This is a prison. This is my house; they should be more understanding. (Participant 18, Year 4)

Admittedly, we do not know the context of these participants' wishes for more counselor understanding. It may be that these participants disliked being held accountable for their behavior in treatment and the dormitory. We are not able to tell this from these data, but future research should consider these possibilities as well as the meaning of "understanding" in the staff-participant relationship, particularly from the participant's perspective.

Finally, two participants felt the Alcoholics Anonymous and Narcotics Anonymous (AA/NA) meetings were unproductive and unhelpful because they were not led by staff. These participants indicated that the lack of leadership and lack of control in the meetings made for unfocused discussions. When asked the part of the program they least liked, two participants said:

[I least liked] AA/NA. There is no staff member present. [The meeting] is led by inmates, and there is usually no control. (Participant 7, Year 1)

[I least liked] the AA part of it; it's not productive. The AA meetings go unsupervised and the inmates do not really want to take control of the meetings. Nothing really gets done. They are a waste of time. (Participant 8, Year 1)

This lack of control and productivity appears to adversely affect other participants' experiences in the program. One participant, who did not specifically discuss the AA/NA meetings, did not like it when other participants disrupted group interactions. He explained:

I hated it when participants were interruptive [sic] in class. They impinged on my ability to learn as well as others. (Participant 4, Year 1)

While only a small segment of the participants participating in the study mentioned the AA/NA meetings as unhelpful, the possibility that participants need more guidance or structure in these meetings is important to consider here and in future research.

CONCLUSION

The purpose of this study was to elicit staff members' and participants' perceptions of a specific prison-based treatment program in one Kentucky prison using in-depth interviews. Several themes emerged in this analysis, including participant motivation, staff-participant communication, race, institutional support, and the frequency of counselor contacts as major areas developed from qualitative interviews. Specifically, staff members and participants generally agreed that the primary motivation for participating in this prison-based substance abuse program was for the early parole opportunity substance abuse program participation provided. The parole opportunity presents a dilemma for prison and program staff since some participants may enter treatment with more motivation to make parole than to participate in substance abuse treatment. However, there are data which support the idea that coerced drug abuse treatment has been successful, particularly in community settings (see Leukefeld et al., 2002). In fact, self-help groups have adopted the saying that involvement comes with time and use the phrase "thirty meetings in thirty days."

Data from this study indicates that staff and participants agreed that at times they sometimes experienced difficulty in communicating with each other. However, despite these communication difficulties both staff and participants described the overall staff-participant relationship as positive. Staff identified race, a lack of institutional support, and understaffing as the main challenges facing the substance abuse treatment program. In a difference in perception, most participants indicated that the two difficulties facing the program included counselors' lack of understanding for participants and the limited opportunities for participants to receive one-on-one counseling. Clearly, the staff-participant contact in both individual and group sessions, with the exception of self-help groups, were generally perceived by participants as positive and helpful. This is an important finding since individual and group sessions are the core of the SAP program. Clearly, increasing the number and intensity of these contacts should be considered.

Findings from this study have implications for providing in-prison substance abuse treatment during incarceration. Administrators and staff should be aware of the potential importance of treatment motivation, participant compliance, and parole. However, once a participant enters treatment, treatment focused on criminal thinking errors (Yochelson & Samenow, 1995) and relapse prevention (Marlatt, 1985) could be beneficial for inmates with substance use issues (Staton et al., 2000). In addition, staff should be aware of the need for participants to maintain one-on-one contact and participation during in-prison treatment, as well as realizing the strains that the prison environment can place on communication between staff and participants. Finally, implications from this study suggest that a mutually supportive and therapeutic environment for treatment should be developed and maintained.

There are limitations to this study which included the purposive selection of participants–both staff and participants. It is also not clear how truthful study participants were since they may have believed that their interview information would be related to their program participation even though strict confidentiality was maintained and consent was given.

With the increase in drug-related offenses which is associated with sentencing provisions, this substance abuse treatment program like other prison-based drug treatment programs focused on changing the drug and criminal behavior of program participants. Evaluation findings (e.g., Inciardi et al., 2002; Wexler et al., 1999) report that prison-based treatment is effective. However, little qualitative data are available to provide in-depth insights into perceptions of treatment. The themes identified in this qualitative study suggest that the program is accomplishing its overall goals. Clearly, correctional administrators as well as prison-based treatment providers should take time to understand and to be aware of similarities and differences in staff and participant perceptions related to motivation, communication, and commitment in order to facilitate the provision of the most effective drug abuse treatment.

REFERENCES

Broome, K. M., Knight, K., Hiller, M. L., & Simpson, D. D. (1996). Drug treatment process indicators for probationers and prediction of recidivism. *Journal of Substance Abuse Treatment, 13*, 487-491.

Charmaz, K. (1983). The grounded theory method: An explication and interpretation. In R. M. Emerson (Ed.), *Contemporary field research: A collection of readings* (pp. 109-126). Prospect Heights, IL: Waveland Press.

Compton, E. R. & Galaway, B. (1994). *Social work processes.* Pacific Grove, CA: Brooks/Cole.

Cronbach, L. J. (1982a). *Designing evaluations of educational and social programs.* San Francisco: Jossey-Bass.

Cronbach, L. J. (1982b). Prudent aspirations for social inquiry. In W. H. Kruskal (Ed.), *The social sciences: Their nature and uses* (pp. 61-81). Chicago: University of Chicago Press.

DeLeon, G. (1988). Legal pressure in therapeutic communities. *Journal of Drug Issues, 18*, 625-640.

Finn, P. (1994). Addressing the needs of cultural minorities in drug treatment. *Journal of Substance Abuse Treatment, 11*, 325-337.

Griffith, J. D., Hiller, M. L., Knight, K. & Simpson, D. D. (1999). A cost-effectiveness analysis of in-prison therapeutic community treatment and risk classification. *The Prison Journal, 79*, 352-368.

Inciardi, J. A., Surratt, H. L., Martin, S. S., & Hooper, R. M. (2002). The importance of aftercare in a corrections-based treatment continuum. In C. G. Leukefeld, F. Tims, & D. Farabee (Eds.), *Treatment of drug offenders: Policies and issues* (pp. 204-216). New York: Springer.

Joe, G. W., Simpson, D. D., & Broome, K. M. (1998). Effects of readiness for drug abuse treatment on participant retention and assessment of process. *Addiction, 93*, 1177-1190.

Lo, C. C. & Stevens, R. C. (2000). Drugs and prisoners: Treatment needs on entering prison. *American Journal on Drug and Alcohol Abuse, 26*, 229-245.

Leukefeld, C. G., Tims, F., & Farabee, D. (2002). *Treatment of drug offenders: Policies and issues.* New York: Springer.

Lofland, J. & Lofland, L. (1995). *Analyzing social settings: A guide to qualitative observation and analysis*. Third Addition. Belmont, CA: Wadsworth.

Marlatt, G. A. (1985). *Relapse prevention: Maintenance strategies in the treatment of addictive behaviors*. New York: Guilford Press.

Martin, S. S., Butzin, C. A., Saum, C. A., & Inciardi, J. A. (1999). Three-year outcomes of therapeutic community treatment for drug-involved offenders in Delaware: From prison to work release to aftercare. *The Prison Journal, 79*, 294-320.

Maynard, D. W. (1996). On "realization" in everyday life: The forecasting of bad news as a social relation. *American Sociological Review, 61*, 109-131.

McCollum, E. E. & Trepper, T. S. (1995). 'Little by little, pulling me through'– Women's perceptions of successful drug treatment: A qualitative inquiry. *Journal of Family Psychotherapy, 6*, 63-82.

McCorkel, J., Harrison, L. D., & Inciardi, J. A. (1998). How treatment is constructed among graduates and dropouts of a prison therapeutic community for women. *Journal of Offender Rehabilitation, 27*, 37-59.

Mead, G. H. (1934). *Mind, self, and society*. Chicago: University of Chicago Press.

Mumola, C. (1999). Substance abuse and treatment, state and federal prisoners, 1997. *Bureau of Justice Statistics Special Report*. Washington, D.C.: U.S. Department of Justice, Office of Justice Programs.

Murdock, S. H., McCoy, C. B., McBride, D. C., & Weppner, R. S. (1980). The social ecology of drug treatment. *Journal of Drug Education, 10*, 49-62.

Simpson, D. D., Joe, G. W., Rowan-Szal, G. A., & Greener, J. M. (1997). Drug abuse treatment process components that improve retention. *Journal of Substance Abuse Treatment, 14*, 565-572.

Staton, M., Leukefeld, C., Logan, T. K., & Purvis, R. (2000). Process evaluation for a prison-based substance abuse program. *Journal of Offender Rehabilitation, 32*, 105-127.

Stephan, J. (1997). *Census of state and federal correctional facilities, 1995*. Washington, D.C.: U.S. Department of Justice, Office of Justice Programs, Bureau of Justice Statistics.

Wexler, H. R., Melnick, G., Lowe, L., & Peters, J. (1999). Three-year reincarceration outcomes for Amity in prison therapeutic community and aftercare in California. *The Prison Journal, 79*, 321-336.

Winick, C. (1990-91). The counselor in drug user treatment. *The International Journal of the Addiictions, 25*, 1479-1502.

Yih-Ing, H. (1995). Drug treatment counselor practices and effectiveness. *Evaluation Review, 19*, 389-408.

Yochelson, S., & Samenow, S. E. (1995). *The criminal personality: A profile for change*. Volume 1. Northvale, NJ: Jason Aronson.

AUTHORS' NOTES

Sarah Goodrum, PhD, is currently an assistant professor in the Department of Anthropology and Sociology at Centre College. Her publications have appeared in *Sociological Inquiry*, *International Encyclopedia of the Social and Behavioral Sciences*, and *Encyclopedia of Criminology and Deviant Behavior*. In other work, she has examined the ways that the criminal justice system and criminal justice professionals influence the recovery of people who had lost a loved one to murder.

Michele Staton, MSW, CSW, is a drug and alcohol project director at the Center on Drug and Alcohol Research at the University of Kentucky. She obtained her BA degree in Psychology from the University of Kentucky in May 1996, and her MSW in December 1998. She is currently working on her PhD. Ms. Staton is currently the study director for a National Institute of Health (NIH)-funded project examining the health service utilization of incarcerated male and female substance abusers. She is also the study director for a National Institute on Drug Abuse (NIDA)-funded project investigating drug court retention through the implementation of an enhanced employment intervention component. Ms. Staton has published in the area of prison-based treatment, women and substance abuse, health service use among incarcerated women, and employment among drug offenders. Her research interests include substance abuse among women, prison-based and substance abuse treatment, health service utilization, and spirituality.

Carl Leukefeld, DSW, is a professor and Chair of Behavioral Science and Director of the Center on Drug and Alcohol Research at the University of Kentucky. He was a commissioned officer and Chief Health Services Officer in the U.S. Public Health Service, and for much of that time he was assigned to the National Institute on Drug Abuse in various management and scientific capacities. He has given presentations and has written articles on treatment, criminal justice, prevention, and AIDS. His current research interests include the use of judicial sanctions, drug abuse treatment, the delivery of rural services, and the impact of HIV on the drug abuser.

J. Matthew Webster, PhD, is an assistant research professor in the Department of Behavioral Science and the Center on Drug and Alcohol Research at the University of Kentucky. His research interests include the physical health, mental health, and risk-taking behaviors of substance abusers. He also serves as a primary evaluator for the interventions of three research studies funded by the National Institute on Drug Abuse and is the study director and a co-principal investigator for the Kentucky DUI project. He contributes to the literature in the areas of substance abuse, criminal justice, and social psychology.

Richard T. Purvis, PsyD, holds a Doctor of Psychology degree in clinical psychology and is Director for the Division of Mental Health for the Department of Corrections. In this capacity, he is responsible for the oversight of the major units within the Division, which provide mental health assessment and treatment services to sexual offenders, substance abusers, seriously mentally ill, and other inmates in need of general mental health intervention. He has been an instructor in a local doctoral psychology program, maintains a small private practice, and performs limited consulting work.

This project is supported by National Institute of Drug Abuse Grant No. R01 DA 11309. The authors thank anonymous reviewers for their comments and suggestions.

Address correspondence to Sarah Goodrum, PhD, Department of Anthropology and Sociology, Centre College, Danville, KY 40422.

☐ *Appendix: Table of Transcript Codes with the Frequency Distribution of the Codes by Interviewee Type, Total, and Use in the Presentation of the Results*

Transcript Code	Administrator	Counselors	Participants	Total	Used
Race	2	5	12	19	9
Gender	2	0	1	3	0
Participant Motivation	2	3	16	21	7
Participant Change	0	0	10	10	0
Staff-Administration Communication	1	3	0	4	0
Staff-Participant Rel./ Comm.	2	5	16	23	10
Participant-to-Participant Comm.	0	0	15	15	2
Program Goals	2	5	12	19	1
Program Challenges[1]	2	5	16	23	13
Program Positives	0	0	8	8	0
Total				145	42

[1] The code "Program Challenges" was sub-divided into two sub-codes: (1) Institutional and Staff Support and (2) Dormitory, Counselors, and Program Meetings, and these two sub-codes in program challenges are presented in the results.

Treating Substance Abusers in Correctional Contexts: New Understandings, New Modalities. Pp. 47-64.
© *2003 by The Haworth Press, Inc. All rights reserved.*
10.1300/J076v37n03_03

Illicit Drug and Injecting Equipment Markets Inside English Prisons: A Qualitative Study

RHIDIAN HUGHES

King's College London

ABSTRACT In recent years, disrupting the supply of illicit drugs and injecting equipment inside Her Majesty's (HM) prisons has become an important focus for prison drug policy. This paper presents findings from qualitative research, which invited 24 drug injectors with prison experience to discuss the role and operation of illicit drug and injecting equipment markets inside prison. These data were obtained from in-depth interviews and small group discussions. The analyses of these findings are grouped under three broad themes. First, why and how drugs and injecting equipment enter prison from outside. Second, the maintenance of supplies inside prison. Third, the availability of drugs and injecting equipment with a special focus on the quality of injecting equipment. These findings raise important implications, not least public health concerns with the transmission of infection. Prison policy should take a much stronger lead in reducing the harms caused by the operation of prison drug and injecting equipment markets. *[Article copies available for a fee from The Haworth Document Delivery Service: 1-800-HAWORTH. E-mail address: <docdelivery@haworthpress.com> Website: <http://www.HaworthPress. com> © 2003 by The Haworth Press, Inc. All rights reserved.]*

KEYWORDS Drugs, drug injectors, injecting equipment, needles, syringes, prison, distribution, networks, markets, risk, infection, human immunodeficiency virus, hepatitis, policy, qualitative research

Large numbers of people are held in Her Majesty's (HM) prisons in England and Wales, and official estimates expect average numbers to rise from an average of 55,300 people in 1996 to 74,500 by the year 2005 (Turner, Gordon, & Powar, 1997). The number of drug offenders has also risen in recent years (Corkery, 1998), and research studies have shown considerable numbers of people dependent on and injecting drugs inside English prisons (Mason, Birmingham, & Grubin, 1997; Brooke, Taylor, Gunn, & Maden, 1998; Edwards, Curtis, & Sherrard, 1999).

The use of illicit drugs in prison has long been a punishable offence, as it has been outside prison. Whilst, the disruption of prison drug markets has always played a role in the operation of the service it was given priority when the Government published a three-year drug strategy, in which one of the objectives was to reduce the supply of drugs and the level of drug use in prison (HM Government, 1995; HM Prison Service, 1995).

Supply control measures include increased perimeter security, the searching of visitors and the provision of lockers for visitors' hand luggage, the use of drug dogs, increased surveillance, including closed-circuit television during visits, the searching of people after visits before they return to the prison wing, and the imposition of "closed visits" for people found to have committed a drugs offence in prison. To reduce the demand for drugs inside prison, strategies include the identification of individuals using drugs through mandatory drug testing, and the provision of treatment, counselling and support.

Given the attention directed towards the role and operation of prison drug and injecting equipment markets inside prison these topics have remained marginal to research agendas. This reflects more widely the formulation of prison drug policies to appease particular ideological concerns with drug use inside prison (Seddon, 1996).

RESEARCH CONTEXT

Drug injectors with prison experience were invited to discuss their understanding of the role and operation of illicit drug and injecting equipment markets inside prisons. These topics were incorporated into a wider study, which examines drug injectors' risk behaviour inside and outside prison. Drug injectors' perspectives of prison life have been explored previously (Hughes & Huby, 2000).

Drug injectors were recruited from two cities in the Northeast of England. Contact was made with drug injectors outside prison with the assistance of services in touch with people who inject drugs. These services include drug agencies, needle and syringe exchange schemes, drop-in centres, probation services and hostels. Snowball sampling techniques together with time spent outside of these settings helped to reach people not in touch with these services.

The ages of the total 24 participants range from between 17 and 36 years and six participants were women. All were white. Participants had spent time inside prison and length of time served on the last occasion in prison ranged from one day to five years. The number of times people had spent in prison, either on remand or on sentence, ranged from one to 18 occasions. At the time of contact 19 people reported "currently" injecting drugs. Participants had been injecting drugs for between nine months and 19 years. Heroin was the first drug of "choice" for 19 people.

In all, 17 in-depth interviews with a vignette (including two pilots) were conducted, as well as three small group discussions comprising respectively five, three and two participants. The length of in-depth interviews ranged from approximately 30 minutes to 150 minutes. Small group discussions ranged from approximately 40 minutes to 120 minutes. These were held in a variety of settings, including service establishments, participants' homes, cafés, pubs and restaurants. All in-depth interviews and small group discussions were tape recorded and fully transcribed verbatim.

To facilitate qualitative data analysis the "Non-numerical Unstructured Data Indexing Searching and Theorizing" software package was used (Qualitative Solutions and Research, 1997). Coding and analysis of data followed established procedures (Miles & Huberman, 1994), which combined prior theoretical knowledge and assumptions with the inductive generation of original concepts and theories (Layder, 1998). Findings are analysed and reported here under three broad themes. First, examining why and how drugs and injecting equipment enter prison from outside. Second, the maintenance of supplies inside prison. Third, the availability of drugs and injecting equipment inside prison with a special focus on the quality of injecting equipment. Slight changes have been made to some participants' extracts only to conceal identities and all names used are fictitious. A brief explanation of drug injectors' vocabulary, as drawn on in this paper, is given in the Appendix.

"GETTING THEM IN": DRUGS AND INJECTING EQUIPMENT ENTERING PRISON

Drugs and injecting equipment are brought into prison to maintain drug dependency and because of a lack of supply networks inside prison. There are two main methods by which drugs and injecting equipment enter prison. First, they are brought in when people enter prison. Second, visitors bring them in.

"Plugging" and "Crutching": Drugs and Injecting Equipment Brought In When Entering Prison

Drugs play an important role in the lives of the drug injectors contacted in this study and this role continues when individuals spend time in prison. The use of drugs can help people to settle in to prison during the early stages, and drug use can also help to break the monotony of mundane prison life. Taking drugs into prison when entering can also be useful in that individuals need not ask others for help to procure supplies. Lorna illustrates this finding:

> I'm going to prison, and it could be for a while and I don't want to get mixed up with the wrong people . . . I take my own drugs in.

Upon entering prison individuals may not have established the necessary social networks that enable drugs and injecting equipment to be procured. Not having a visitor to bring in supplies through visits was one important reason for bringing drugs and injecting equipment into prison when entering. As Jane reports:

> I'd finished with the boyfriend who was a dealer so I didn't have anyone to bring anything up for me and I knew I was going down. . . . When I went to court that morning I got a teenth and a half and plugged it and I got a pin, I took a pin in with me.

Drugs and injecting equipment can be brought in when people enter prison from outside either at the onset of imprisonment or upon return from a temporary release period. People resident in lower security establishments may also work outside the prison and in these cases deposits at strategic locations placed there by friends and family enable people to obtain drugs and injecting equipment. People are searched on entering prison so it is difficult to conceal supplies on the person within clothing. Instead items can be concealed in the anus or vagina. As Lewis said:

> I've known somebody whose got all his gear, citric, needles, even a little spoon, bent it round, put it in a Smarty tube in a Durex and up his bum.

The Council of Europe (1995) emphasises the need for drug injectors to observe the rules of hygiene. From the outset, however, drugs and injecting equipment clearly enter prison through unhygienic activities. Drug injectors explained that injecting equipment is more difficult to conceal than drugs inside the body. Smuggling personal sets of injecting equipment into prison may help to prevent individuals sharing injecting equipment, subsequently reducing their risk of infection through this route. However, bringing complete sets of injecting equipment into prison is not easy and sometimes only a needle may be brought in; other injecting equipment will need to be obtained inside prison, usually involving sharing.

"Taking a Visit": Drugs and Injecting Equipment Brought In During Visits

Unless people spend only a short period of time in prison supplies need to be maintained in order to avoid drug withdrawal. Visits play an important role in the maintenance of drug supplies. Contacts from outside prison assist by passing drugs and injecting equipment to people during visits. This section reports first on the planning and preparation and second on the visit and the exchange of drugs and injecting equipment.

"Getting Ready": Planning and Preparation

Making contact with people outside prison, typically by letter or telephone, allows drug injectors to ask for drugs and injecting equipment, albeit subtly. Keith describes the way he went about this:

> I got a letter saying he was coming up on a visit . . . I said . . . "are you going to bring me a present and a prick." And he's thinking "a parcel of smack and a works," and that's what he brought up for me.

Drug injectors identified a number of informal rules in prison, many of which reflect the need to remain inconspicuous. When expecting a visit it was important to maintain secrecy. Martin illustrates this on the basis of other people's experiences:

> That's a rule you don't tell a single soul when you're getting a visit. Sometimes I've heard people getting caught on their visits because their pad-mate's talking to his girlfriend on the phone "it's all right love, my pad-mate is getting a visit and he will be coming up with this that and the other." It's recorded on the phone and then they come and nick you.

When information such as this is obtained by prison officers it should be documented in a security report that, if deemed reliable, is acted upon. Some individuals suspected of bringing in drugs and injecting equipment might be placed under increased observation. When individuals believe they are under observation, strategies to avoid detection may be employed, which can include cancelling the supply. Jane illustrates this:

> If I thought that I was going to get searched and it was on top for me. Say like the night before I got a visit, yeah, something happened that was a bit on top. Our wing was getting searched or whatever or they had suspicion that I was using I'd phone my visitor and tell them not to bring any works up or any scag up.

In situations such as these people may try to find someone else to take a visit for them. As Martin said:

> You get someone else to take a visit for ya at the same time. Your missis meets them outside the gaol at the same time, gives them the parcel and then they pass it through on their visit.

Thus, considerable planning and preparation is necessary for a visit. The outcome of a visit is, however, dependent on the actual exchange.

"Pass Them On": The Prison Visit

Visitors to prison need to conceal drugs and injecting equipment to ensure they are not discovered during routine security searches and may conceal drugs inside the body. Visitors may also use other techniques to conceal drugs and injecting equipment. Jane describes her experiences:

> Well I had someone bring my daughter up and they put them in my daughter's nappy. Not while my daughter was wearing it, but in a spare nappy. So I undid the lining and put them in and they don't show up on the scanner you see 'cos they're blocked in with cotton wool inside the nappy, you see, so I had a supply of clean works . . . I was asking them to bring five in a week.

Other methods include storage in the mouth and passing drugs when kissing. As Karen said:

> You can smuggle them in by kissing and stuff and just pass them on. And you can just hide them at the back of your filling. So it's really easy to get them in.

Once drugs have been exchanged the recipient conceals them. Drugs may also be swallowed although this can be the least favoured method because of the time taken for drugs to pass through the body and because people often want drugs immediately. Alternatively, if drugs are swallowed, people may induce vomiting when back on the prison wing rather than wait for the drugs to pass through the body. Drugs may be concealed in the anus, vagina, mouth and throat. These methods are considered more favourable when larger amounts of drugs, which are difficult to swallow, are being brought in. As Natasha reports:

> He [visitor] used to put it in his mouth and spit it in a cup and I used to either swallow it and puke it back up or crutch it depending on. So I'd have it in my mouth, I'd take a drink, spit it out and five minutes later, I'd get the drink and put it in my mouth. . . . Sometimes you can keep it in the side of your mouth but it is quite a big lump so you have to crutch it.

Concealing drugs in the anus or vagina is a difficult task but can be made easier having made certain preparations. Injecting equipment was recognised as more difficult to conceal than drugs. Consequently needles without a syringe barrel would be brought in during visits. As Robert said:

> She [partner] brought a couple of needles up with her but she couldn't exactly bring the works, you know, to smuggle them in would be hard.

Drug injectors are reliant on other people for the provision of sterile injecting equipment. This reliance can mean that there is little choice over the equipment received and there is no guarantee that it is sterile.

Prison visits take place in a very closely observed environment, which is increasingly assisted with closed-circuit television. If prison visitors and residents are caught there are a number of punishments that may be imposed. Prison visitors face arrest. Prison residents face serving additional days on a sentence, being segregated, and having no-contact visits. The threat of being caught can make exchanging drugs an unnerving experience as Karen explains:

> They've got cameras on each side of the room. There's about four cameras and beside officers watching you. You are allowed to kiss and that but they are going to be watching you. You don't want to make the mistake of dropping it out of your mouth. And so basically you had to be careful how you did it. It was nerve racking.

Some people are caught attempting to supply drugs and injecting equipment into prison. This may be when planning and preparation ahead of the visit has been inadequate and when individuals are placed under observation. Lorna attempted an exchange whilst under observation but was caught and punished:

> I got a visit I was put on the obs table and put on top and they got it off me. So I went down the block for seven days.

Despite the problems, some people reported regularly receiving drugs and injecting equipment through visits. For other people supplies were more sporadic, often depending on visitors' contacts with drug suppliers in the community. Friends, family and sexual partners would procure supplies, but not everyone could succeed. Some people could obtain drugs more readily then others. Karen's sister was able to supply her with drugs:

> Me sister . . . she knows one of the dealers. She just gets it in for me if I ask her to.

Thus, the exchange of drugs and injecting equipment occurs despite the threat of being caught and punished.

"YOU GET NOTHING FOR NOTHING INSIDE": MAINTAINING SUPPLIES OF DRUGS AND INJECTING EQUIPMENT INSIDE PRISON

A number of factors influence the exchange of drugs and injecting equipment inside prison. The following were identified as particularly important in the present study: trading and giving of drugs and injecting equipment, credit and debt, and theft.

"You Just Do a Deal": Trading and Giving of Drugs and Injecting Equipment

Ownership of drugs and injecting equipment can confer a privileged position inside prison. It enables owners to levy a charge to others for the use of injecting equipment and, similarly, the trade of drugs for the loan of injecting equipment. These findings were located within a wider prison culture that asserts, "you get nothing for nothing inside." Lorna illustrates this:

> There's no point in lending it for nothing is there. If she could end up with something. . . . She wouldn't just give her them for nothing. What's the point?

Drugs are usually traded for a loan of injecting equipment. The form drugs are traded in varies. A small bag of drugs may be obtained for the receiver to prepare for injection themselves. During the process of preparing drugs for injection, drugs are liquefied and measures of this liquid may be traded. When more than one set of injecting equipment is available this process may occur through syringe-mediated syringe-sharing (Grund, Friedman, Stern, Jose, Neaigus, Curtis, & Des Jarlais, 1996). The filter used during the process of drug injecting contains drugs, which may also be passed on. With the exception of trading a bag of drugs, these trading practices constitute infection risk.

The trading of drugs for injecting equipment varies depending on a range of factors, such as whether the owner of the injecting equipment needs drugs themselves. Injecting equipment would be loaned for a limited time period or for a small number of drug injections. If a suitable trade was not offered, or was considered unsatisfactory, then injecting equipment might not be lent out. Colin explains:

> He'd charge him to use the works. Unless he comes up with a price he wouldn't use the works. No one used our works without 'cos like they weren't coming up with a price. Well a couple of people did, well, come up with a price but a lot of people wouldn't come up with a price.

Trading led to the sharing of resources, including the sharing of injecting equipment. As Keith reports:

> You've got the gear, I've got the works. I've got no gear right. I'll lend you my works if you give me a wash-out of your gear. Like both ways. You need what I've got, I need what you've got. You just do a deal.

Drugs and injecting equipment were the main currency but other items included tobacco, telephone cards and, less commonly reported, money. Women reported trading other personal items, such as shampoo and soap. In addition to the trading of tangible assets, services may also be traded for drugs and injecting equipment. As Lorna notes:

> They might want you to work for them listening to what goes on and who brings things in. And then getting someone to take the drugs off them. Running about for them.

Thus, people usually trade drugs and injecting equipment in order that both parties benefit from the trade to some extent. However, a distinction can be made here with giving based more on the principles of reciprocity. People who are undergoing drug withdrawal or have recently entered prison may be freely provided with drugs as Karen illustrates:

> *Karen:* Sometimes when you first come in people, you know, to sort you out they just give you some for nothing and you don't have to pay them back. But after the first time you've got to start fending for yourself. So it's not too bad.
> *Researcher:* Why do you think they give you stuff for the first time?
> *Karen:* I don't know. Maybe it's because when they came in they were rattling the same as anyone else. Maybe they knew somebody who maybe gave them a fix for the first time. Because like everyone goes through it. So it's just helping people out until you're on your feet really.

This extract shows how drug injectors do not like to see others experiencing drug withdrawal and in need of drug injection. In these situations, people may be helped, especially during the early period of settling into prison and this may be influenced by the extent of social closeness and distance between individuals (Hughes, 2000a). They also engender future obligations should the giver ever be in need of drugs so that communal giving in this way may be understood as a form of social insurance. It is in drug injectors' interests, individually and collectively, that communal distribution activities continue to take place in order that future supplies of drugs and injecting equipment are secured. Martin illustrates an example of communal distribution of injecting equipment:

I'd go on the phone but hide it [injecting equipment] where the telephone is. Then the next lad goes to the phone booth and that how we used to.

Thus, drugs and injecting equipment may be directly traded for tangible assets and services. Giving may occur with fewer obligations being met at the time of the exchange. However, trading and giving may engender, implicitly or explicitly, future obligations. This may constitute credit and associated with this is the problem of debt.

"Lay Ons" and "Debtheads": Credit and Debt

Drugs can be provided on credit. Generally most people reported that drugs were not provided in this way. Others suggest, however, that credit was more likely to occur amongst the socially close. Jake explains:

They won't do lay ons unless you're fairly good mates with the person selling the drugs and they'll know that you'll actually pay for it.

Prisons are heterogeneous and credit strategies differ between prisons. Don suggests that credit is more common in prisons holding people on a long-term basis, where there has been more time for social closeness to develop. As Don said:

You've got people doing life, like no less than five years basically and the people in there are like big dealers. And they can get hold of a lot of drugs. They will lay it on. You can go to hundreds of pounds of debt. They know you are not going no-where because you're doing that many years.

Credit can lead to debt inside prison with far-reaching consequences. Jane reports:

He is going to get himself into worse shit by taking scag because he is going to owe them and they'll always remember that and keep on his case for it.

There can be violent sanctions directed towards debtors, which may, ultimately, result in debtors being placed on a protected prison regime. The threat of violence inside prison also permeates the theft of drugs and injecting equipment.

"Taxing": Theft

Inside prison drugs, like anything else, are at risk of being stolen. The likelihood of drugs and injecting equipment being stolen depends on their availability and desirability. In an attempt to reduce the risk of theft, drugs and injecting equipment may be concealed inside the body. However, if it is known that an individual possesses drugs, these drugs may be physically removed. Assaults of this kind have also been reported elsewhere (Devlin, 1998). As Dan said:

> Say you got a visit and someone knew you had scored, well, you know, the whole gaol will know. They would ask you for a sorter and if you didn't give it I've heard of people getting a toothbrush and taking it up someone's arse and scraping the gear out.

It is important, therefore, for knowledge of possession of drugs and injecting equipment to be kept to a minimum. As few people as possible should know about the possession of drugs and injecting equipment as Lorna reflects:

> I had a girl come up to me and say I can get you some works. [I said], "let me talk to my pad-mate about it." She [pad-mate] says, "well I don't think there are any works in prison so obviously what she'd do is tell you she can get you some works in prison and when you ask for them she is going to know that you've got something and she'll tax ya."

Remaining inconspicuous inside prison is important to avoid drawing attention, which risks violence. The theft of drugs and injecting equipment from individuals represents a real threat to drug injectors when they spend time inside prison. It is also important to recognise that the theft of drugs and injecting equipment is closely related to their availability.

"THEY'RE AROUND": AVAILABILITY OF DRUGS AND INJECTING EQUIPMENT INSIDE PRISONS

The availability of drugs and injecting equipment varies and depends on, for example, the reliability of security information and associated enforcement activities together with the degree of drug injectors' success in bringing drugs into prison when entering and making exchanges during visits. The following subsections report first on the availability of drugs and second on the availability of injecting equipment, including a special focus on the quality of the latter.

"Keeping a Habit in Gaol": Availability of Drugs

Some people were able to procure drugs in prison with few problems. Terry attributed his ability to procure drugs to his relationship with a number of suppliers:

There was like four of my dealers in there. They were on remand so they got visits every day so the supply was really brilliant, better than waiting on the street corner. You know, just walking up one landing and sorted, you were off.

The relational dynamic that underpins drug availability is important. Drugs may be easier to procure amongst the socially close (Hughes, 2000c). Lower drug availability was reported when people did not know others and when drug-using activities were particularly clandestine. As Lorna said:

You don't get much drugs in there and if you do no-one will declare.

The variable and limited drug supplies can make drug dependency difficult to maintain. Colin notes:

There's no keeping a habit in gaol because you don't know when it's going to come and when it's not going to come.

The quantities of drug sold were generally smaller, sometimes by half, inside prison compared to what would be received outside prison for the same price. Inhaling these smaller quantities of drugs inside prison can be insufficient to sustain drug dependency. Consequently, drug injection is preferred, providing a much stronger drug administration. The limited availability of drugs inside prison may contribute to a shift in drug taking behaviour towards drug injecting. Individuals may, therefore, be confronted with situations where they may be called upon to share injecting equipment. Craig reported only injecting drugs inside prison, when outside prison he switched back to inhaling drugs:

The bags in there were nothing like out here so you couldn't smoke it on foil, you had to inject to get enough off a tenner, you know. Five phone cards otherwise if you were putting it on foil you were spending like 100 pound a day at least.

Thus, for some people prisons may alter drug-using behaviour. The findings presented here can help to understand why some people inject for the first time inside prisons (Gore, Bird, & Ross, 1995; Taylor, Goldberg, Emslie, Wrench, Gruer, Cameron, Black, Davis, McGregor, Follett, Harvey, Basson, & McGavigan, 1995) and why prisons may contribute to sustained risk behaviour. Furthermore, these findings can illustrate why some drug injectors may perceive prison to be a greater risk environment than outside (Power, Marková, McKee, & Kilfedder, 1996). When an individual's desire for drugs is reduced as a result of, for example, limited availability and having undergone drug withdrawal, then the use and injection of drugs may be reduced so that prisons can also help to hinder drug-injecting behaviour. Tim said:

> I did enquire to see if there was anything on the wing and someone like filled me in on [what] the size of the bags were like in prison. Thought about it then thought, "it is not worth bothering with."

"There's Only a Few Works on the Landing":
Availability of Injecting Equipment

Some people reported not being able to locate injecting equipment. This could reflect a lack of supplies or that individuals were outside these social networks where drug-injecting equipment was available. This can reinforce the need to bring injecting equipment when entering prison as discussed earlier. Sharon said:

> I couldn't get hold of one [set of injecting equipment]. It was too hard, really hard, to get hold of one.

Other people reported some limited availability of injecting equipment. As a consequence injecting equipment would be shared. Kieran reports:

> There's only a few works on the landing you normally have to share because it is hard getting them in.

However, other people may not need to share when regular visits ensure a steady supply. Mark reports:

> I was on remand for a few months and I had a friend visiting me and was fetching me works when I wanted them so I was OK and I had my own works all the time I was in so I didn't need to share.

Outside prison the unsafe disposal of used injecting equipment represents a serious public health risk and reducing this risk remains a future challenge for policy (Neale, 1998). Outside prison needles and syringes are disposed of in a number of ways and are not often used for more than a small number of drug injections. Inside prison the reverse can apply. Injecting equipment may represent capital and it is less likely to be disposed of voluntarily. There are situations, however, when injecting equipment may be disposed of inside prison. For people who received a regular supply of injecting equipment, used injecting equipment would sometimes be passed on to others. Surplus injecting equipment may also be traded. Some individuals reported keeping one set of injecting equipment for personal use and another for communal exchange. Other individuals reported freely passing on used injecting equipment. The disposal of injecting equipment may also occur in ways that result in individuals having no need to share other injecting equipment that has been set aside specifically for personal use. Mark said:

> On my first visit I got another one so the one I already had I passed that on, "you can have that."

In contrast, injecting equipment may be lent to others on the condition that it is returned, which may be part of trade relations and reciprocal exchanges discussed earlier. Some people also reported injecting equipment being bought and sold. However, there can be little guarantee of its sterility. A discussion with Kieran illustrates these issues:

> *Kieran:* I got one clean needle but I bought that off someone.
> *Researcher:* Was it sterile, in a pack then?
> *Kieran:* No, but he said it was clean. I'm sure it was clean.

The quality of injecting equipment varied from the new to the old. Injecting equipment inside prison would be used for an extended period because of limited and variable supplies. To maintain injecting equipment, needles are sharpened on walls and match boxes. After continual use injecting equipment was described as, "old and scabby" and "bodged up." Drug injectors described very poor quality needles. Terry explains:

> When they've been used that many times the actual fine point seems to go like a hook. If you run it across your finger you can feel it pulling your skin or if you rub it on your nail you'll see it score your nail.

In this instance, Terry goes on to explain the problems of using these poor quality needles:

> You could do some damage once it's inside because again when you're withdrawing it you feel it pull, you know, like catching a fish sort of thing.

When needle and syringe sets are incomplete, missing items would be substituted from other needle and syringe sets or from materials available inside prison. As Tim describes:

> People using, you know, the inside of a pen, you know, what the actual ink is in. Cleaning it out, sharpening it up and using that to inject.

Poor quality injecting equipment has also been noted in other prison studies (Turnbull, Stimson, & Stillwell, 1994; Taylor, 1996). Notwithstanding the serious risk of infection, drug injectors are at more risk of health complications, including scarring and bruising, abscesses and thrombosis from using extremely poor quality injecting equipment (Morrison, Elliott, & Gruer, 1997).

The lack of sterile injecting equipment inside prison creates a need for drug injectors to repeatedly use injecting equipment, which raises serious concerns regarding the spread of infection. Drug injectors recognise the risk of infection but still put themselves at risk despite the grim drug injecting environment. Even though drug injectors considered it necessary to clean injecting equipment prior to sharing, this was generally perceived to be undertaken less effectively inside prison compared with outside prison (Hughes, 2000c).

CONCLUDING DISCUSSION AND POLICY IMPLICATIONS

The research presented in this paper has demonstrated how prison drugs and injecting equipment markets play an important role in drug injectors' lives when they spend time inside prison. These markets operate with determined efforts on the part of individuals and groups. Drug-injecting activities inside prison are clandestine, and involve considerable planning and organisation.

Current prison drug policy attempts to disrupt drug and injecting equipment supply networks and provide drug treatment (HM Prison Service, 1998b). However, successive prison drug strategies (HM Prison Service, 1995; 1998b) have been introduced partially. There is an overemphasis on disrupting supply networks with much less attention being given to drug treatment and harm reduction measures. This discrepancy may be due, in part, to prison drug budgets being provided at the same time as a cut in overall prison spending. Consequently, the drug budget subsidises the overall prison budget cut resulting in fewer drug treatment places (The Observer, 15th August 1999: 27).

Drug injectors' responses to limited availability of drugs and injecting equipment mean that drugs and injecting equipment enter prisons usually concealed inside the body to minimise discovery by prison staff. These methods are contrary to Council of Europe (1995) recommendations that encourage drug injectors to observe basic rules of hygiene with regards to drug injecting inside prison.

Once drugs are brought into prison, strategies to maintain drug-injecting activities usually centre on the exchange of drugs for injecting equipment or vice versa. A distinction is apparent between drugs and injecting equipment that are directly traded and where giving takes place with less emphasis on immediate returns. Direct trading and giving, however, involve the shared use of resources. Within this trading context it is important to promote safer injecting practices in order to minimise infection spread via the use of shared injecting equipment.

Reciprocal giving of drugs and injecting equipment, the provision of drugs on credit and associated problems with debt, and the theft of drugs demonstrate how prison drug and injecting equipment markets prosper on limited resources and cause a great deal of harm. It highlights the need for policies to take serious steps to reduce drug-related harm inside prison. Equally, various forms of injecting equipment sharing have been identified. These issues raise serious public health concerns regarding the transmission of infection. To reduce infection risk it is essential that drug injectors inside prison are provided with sterile injecting equipment on an exchange basis (Hughes, 2000d).

Beyond these issues, there is the need for policy to adopt a wider perspective when responding to drug use in prison. Drug use and drug dependency does not occur in a vacuum inside prison. Drug use is, at least partly, the product of a oppressive prison regime where drugs are used in a desperate attempt to combat boredom and isolation (Hughes & Huby, 2000). A holistic policy approach should aim to, among other things, tackle the reasons why drug injectors enter prison; how their imprisonment can be reduced; why drug injectors' need for illicit drugs is sustained in prison; and how integrated drug treatment strategies, including the provision of substitute drugs, can be forged between prison and the wider community. The development of a prison drug policy seriously committed to minimising the problems associated with drug injection inside prison, including a reduction in punitive drug control measures, could, potentially, reduce the harm presently associated with prison drug and injecting equipment markets.

REFERENCES

Brooke, D., Taylor, C., Gunn, J., & Maden, A. (1998). Substance misusers remanded to prison–a treatment opportunity? *Addiction*, 93(12), 1851-1856.

Corkery, J.M. (1998). *Statistics of Drug Seizures and Offenders Dealt With, United Kingdom, 1996* (Home Office Statistical Bulletin, Issue 10/98). London: Government Statistical Service.

Council of Europe. (1995). *Prison and Criminological Aspects of the Control of Transmissible Diseases Including Aids and Related Health Problems in Prisons: Recommendation No. R (93) 6 and Explanatory Report*. Strasbourg: Council of Europe Press.

Devlin, A. (1998). *What's Wrong with Women's Prisons*. Winchester: Waterside Press.

Edwards, A., Curtis, S., & Sherrard, J. (1999). Survey of risk behaviour and HIV prevalence in an English prison. *International Journal of STD and AIDS*, 10(7), 464-466.

Gore, S.M., Bird, A.G., & Ross, A. (1995). Prison rites: Starting to inject inside. *British Medical Journal*, 311(7013), 1135-1136.

Grund, J-P.C., Friedman, S.R., Stern, L.S., Jose, B., Neaigus, A., Curtis, R., & Des Jarlais, D.C. (1996). Syringe-mediated drug sharing among injecting drug users: Patterns, social context and implications for transmission of blood-borne pathogens. *Social Science and Medicine*, 42(5), 691-703.

HM Government. (1995). *Tackling Drugs Together: A Strategy for England 1995-98* (Cm 2846). London: HM Stationery Office.

HM Government. (1998). *Tackling Drugs to Build a Better Britain: The Government's 10-Year Strategy for Tackling Drug Misuse* (Cm 3945). London: Stationery Office.

HM Prison Service. (1995). *Drug Misuse in Prison.* London: HM Prison Service.

HM Prison Service. (1998a). *The Review of the Prison Service Drug Strategy, "Drug Misuse in Prison."* London: HM Prison Service.

HM Prison Service. (1998b). *Tackling Drugs in Prison: The Prison Service Drug Strategy.* London: HM Prison Service.

Hughes, R. (2000a). Drug injectors and prison mandatory drug testing. *Howard Journal of Criminal Justice*, 39(1), 1-13.

Hughes, R. (2000b) "Friendships are a big part of it": Social relationships, social distance and HIV risks. *Substance Use and Misuse*, 35(9), 1149-1176.

Hughes, R.A. (2000c). Drug injectors and the cleaning of needles and syringes. *European Addiction Research*, 6(1), 20-30.

Hughes, R.A. (2000d). Lost opportunities? Prison needle and syringe exchange. *Drugs: Education, Prevention, and Policy*, 7(1), 75-86.

Hughes, R., & Huby, M. (2000). Life in prison: Perspectives of drug injectors. *Deviant Behavior*, 21(5), 451-479.

Layder, D. (1998). *Sociological Practice: Linking Theory and Social Research.* London: Sage.

Mason, D., Birmingham, L., & Grubin, D. (1997). Substance use in remand prisoners: A consecutive case study. *British Medical Journal*, 315(7099), 8-21.

Miles, M.B., & Huberman, A.M. (1994). *Qualitative Data Analysis: An Expanded Sourcebook* (Second Edition). London: Sage.

Morrison, A., Elliott, L., & Gruer, L. (1997). Injecting-related harm and treatment-seeking behaviour among injecting drug users. *Addiction*, 92(10), 1349-1352.

Neale, J. (1998). Reducing risks: Drug users' views of accessing and disposing of injecting equipment. *Addiction Research*, 6(2), 147-163.

Power, K.G., Marková, I., McKee, K.J., & Kilfedder, C. (1996). Correlates of HIV/AIDS knowledge in a Scottish prison sample. *Health Education Research*, 11(3), 287-297.

Qualitative Solutions and Research. (1997). *NUD*IST 4 User Guide.* Melbourne: Qualitative Solutions and Research.

Rutter, S., Dolan, K., Wodak, A., Hall, W., Maher, L., & Dixon, D. (1995). *Is Syringe Exchange Feasible in a Prison Setting? An Exploratory Study of the Issues* (Technical Report Number 25). Sydney: National Drug and Alcohol Research Centre.

Seddon, T. (1996). Drug control in prison. *The Howard Journal of Criminal Justice*, 35(4), 327-335.

Taylor, A. (1996). Drug use and injecting behaviour in Glenochil prison. In N. Squires & J. Strobl (Eds.), *Healthy Prisons: A Vision for the Future*, pp. 176-180. Liverpool: University of Liverpool, Department of Public Health.

Taylor, A., Goldberg, D.J, Emslie, J., Wrench, J., Gruer, L., Cameron, S., Black, J., Davis, B., McGregor, J., Follett, E., Harvey, J., Basson, J., & McGavigan, J. (1995). Outbreak of HIV infection in a Scottish prison. *British Medical Journal*, 310(6975), 289-292.

Turnbull, P.J., Stimson, G.V., & Stillwell, G. (1994). *Drug Use in Prison.* Horsham: AIDS Education and Research Trust.

Turner, D., Gordon, S., & Powar, I. (1997). *Projections of Long Term Trends in the Prison Population to 2005.* London: Government Statistical Service.

AUTHOR'S NOTE

Rhidian Hughes, DPhil, is Senior Research Fellow at Guy's, King's and St. Thomas' School of Medicine, King's College London. His research interests are in the areas of social policy, palliative care, health, illicit drug use, criminal justice and research methodology.

The author would like to thank all the participants and the services that helped in recruitment for this study. Also to Dr. Meg Huby for her encouragement and support for this work throughout.

Address correspondence to Rhidian Hughes, DPhil, Guy's, King's and St. Thomas' School of Medicine, Kings College London, Third Floor, The Weston Education Centre, Cutcombe Road, Denmark Hill, London, SE5 9RJ, United Kingdom (E-mail: rhidian.hughes@ukonline.co.uk).

APPENDIX

Explanatory Notes on Drug Injectors' Vocabulary

"Bags":	Parcels of drugs.
"Block":	Segregation.
"Citric":	Citric acid.
"Crutch":	Concealment in vagina.
"Debtheads":	Debtors.
"Dope":	Cannabis.
"Durex":	Condom.
"Fanny":	Vagina.
"Fix":	Drug injection.
"Gear":	Heroin.
"Geezer":	Man.
"Habit":	Drug dependence.
"Lay on":	Credit advance.
"Obs":	Observation.
"Pad-mate":	Other occupant(s) of prison cell.
"Pin":	Needle.
"Plug":	Concealment in anus.
"Pooh":	Faeces.
"Puke":	Vomit.
"Scag":	Heroin.
"Score":	Procure drugs.
"Screws":	Prison officers.
"Smack":	Heroin.
"Smackheads":	Heroin users.
"Sort":	Procure drugs.
"Taxing":	Theft or extortion.
"Teenth":	Sixteenth of an ounce of drugs.
"Wash-out":	Residue drugs in a filter can be dehydrated and reheated to produce a further injection.
"Works":	Needle and syringe.

Treating Substance Abusers in Correctional Contexts: New Understandings, New Modalities. Pp. 65-94.
10.1300/J076v37n03_04

Multiple Measures of Outcome in Assessing a Prison-Based Drug Treatment Program

MICHAEL L. PRENDERGAST

University of California, Los Angeles

ELIZABETH A. HALL

University of California, Los Angeles

HARRY K. WEXLER

National Development and Research Institutes

ABSTRACT Evaluations of prison-based drug treatment programs typically focus on one or two dichotomous outcome variables related to recidivism. In contrast, this paper uses multiple measures of outcomes related to crime and drug use to examine the impact of prison treatment. Crime variables included self-report data of time to first illegal activity, arrest type, and number of months incarcerated. Days to first reincarceration and type of reincarceration are based on official records. Drug use variables included self-report data of the time to first use and drug testing results. Prisoners randomly assigned to treatment performed significantly better than controls on: days to first illegal activity, days to first incarceration, days to first use, type of reincarceration, and mean number of months incarcerated. No differences were found in type of first arrest or in drug test results. Subjects who completed both prison-based and community-based treatment performed significantly better than subjects who received lesser amounts of treatment on every measure. Survival analysis suggested that subjects were most vulnerable to recidivism in the 60 days after release. Although the overall results from the analyses presented support the effectiveness of prison-based treatment, conclusions about the effectiveness of a treatment program may vary depending on which outcomes are selected. The results of this study argue for including more rather than fewer outcomes in assessing the impact of prison-based substance abuse treatment. *[Article copies available for a fee from The Haworth Document Delivery Service: 1-800-HAWORTH. E-mail address: <docdelivery@haworthpress.com> Website: <http://www.HaworthPress.com>* © *2003 by The Haworth Press, Inc. All rights reserved.]*

KEYWORDS Recidivism, prisons, parole, drug abuse, outcome assessment

DRUG ABUSE TREATMENT IN PRISONS

Beginning in the late 1980s, state and federal initiatives began to address the severe demands imposed on the criminal justice system by substance-abusing offenders. In 1988, the Federal Bureau of Prisons began development of a broad and comprehensive system of prison-based treatment programs, transitional services, and outpatient programs for offenders under its jurisdiction (Murray, 1996). Beginning in the late 1980s, Project REFORM, funded by the Bureau of Justice Assistance, and later Project RECOVERY, funded by the Center for Substance Abuse Treatment, provided technical assistance to 20 states in planning and developing substance abuse programming for prisoners with substance abuse problems (Wexler, 1997). The annual National Drug Control Strategy, prepared by the Office of National Drug Control Policy (1997, 1998, 1999), has encouraged the development of treatment and rehabilitation services for drug-using offenders (e.g., Treatment Accountability for Safer Communities [formerly Treatment Alternatives to Street Crime], drug court programs, prison treatment programs). The Residential Substance Abuse Treatment for State Prisoners Formula Grant Program, one of the provisions of the Violent Crime Control and Law Enforcement Act of 1994, authorized funding for states to develop comprehensive approaches to providing treatment for substance-abusing offenders, including intensive programs for inmates and relapse prevention training. As a result of these efforts, many state prison systems established prison- and parole-based drug treatment programs during the 1990s (Camp & Camp, 1998).

As part of the growth of prison-based treatment, the original therapeutic community (TC) treatment model was modified and adapted to correctional environments, becoming the major modality for treating substance abusers in prison (Inciardi et al., 1997; Knight, Simpson, & Hiller, 1999; Martin, Butzin, Saum, & Inciardi, 1999; Wexler, 1994; Wexler, Blackmore, & Lipton, 1991; Wexler, DeLeon et al., 1999; Wexler & Lipton, 1993; Wexler, Melnick et al.,

1999). Prison-based TC treatment assumes that the drug problems characteristic of most inmates require high-intensity treatment designed to restructure the attitudes and thinking of participants and to instill the social functioning and relapse prevention skills that would help inmates improve their adjustment in the community on parole (Wexler, 1995a). Increasingly, prison TC programs are followed by treatment in community-based programs in order to reinforce and consolidate the gains made in prison programs (Inciardi, 1996).

REVIEW OF EXISTING EVALUATIONS

The results from early evaluations of prison-based TC programs in several states have provided support for the development of such prison programs nationwide. The program evaluations that have received the most attention are those conducted at Stay'n Out in New York, Cornerstone in Oregon, KEY/ CREST in Delaware, New Vision in Texas, Forever Free and Amity in California, and the Federal Bureau of Prison programs. Findings from these program evaluations are summarized below (the Amity results appear in a later section). Only findings on outcome differences between treatment and comparison groups are summarized.

The evaluation of the Stay'n Out prison TC in New York, conducted by researchers at NDRI (Wexler, Falkin, & Lipton, 1990), has probably had the greatest impact on correctional treatment policy and programming. Established in the late 1970s, Stay'n Out provided treatment at both men's and women's correctional facilities. Using a quasi-experimental design, the authors found that, over a 40-month period, the TC was more effective than no treatment or than other types of less intensive treatment in reducing recidivism. Specifically, the percentage of men TC participants who were rearrested (27%) was significantly lower than that for men in two less intensive treatment groups (35% for the milieu group, 40% for the counseling group) and for men in the no-treatment comparison group (41%). Statistically significant differences among the four groups were not found for time to arrest or for positive parole discharge. No statistically significant differences were found for women.

In an evaluation of Cornerstone, a TC program in the Oregon prison system established in 1975, Field (1985) compared all Cornerstone clients who graduated between 1976 and 1979 with dropouts from the program and with a sample of Oregon parolees who did not receive treatment. Three years after release, 71% of the program graduates had *not* been reincarcerated, compared with 26% of the dropouts and 63% of the parolee sample. Similarly, while over one-half (54%) of the graduates had *not* been convicted of any crime over the 3-year period, this was true for only 15% of the dropouts and 36% of the parolee sample. In a second study of Cornerstone, Field (1992) compared recidivism among Cornerstone graduates with three dropout groups defined by decreasing time in the program. Although 63% of the graduates were rearrested, 49% of them were convicted of a new offense, and 26% were reincarcerated. By comparison, 79% of clients in treatment for more than six months were rearrested, 72% were convicted, and 63% were reincarcerated. For those who stayed in treatment for less than two months, 92% were rearrested, 89% were convicted, and 85% were reincarcerated.

The evaluations of the Stay'n Out and Cornerstone programs did not consider the contribution to outcomes of community treatment for program graduates after release to parole. Recent evaluations of prison TCs have indicated that adding community treatment significantly improves clients' behavior while under parole supervision. For instance, the New Vision program in Kyle, Texas, is a nine-month in-prison TC, followed by a three-month stay in a community residential treatment center. A 12-month follow-up study indicated that 18% of clients who participated in both the prison TC and the community residential program were rearrested or reincarcerated, compared with 29% of those who participated in the prison TC only and 33% of those who were in the no-treatment control group (Knight, Simpson, Chatham, & Camacho, 1997).

The evaluation of the KEY/CREST program in Delaware also tested the effects of enhancing the in-prison treatment experience with treatment while under community supervision. KEY is a prison-based TC for male inmates with histories of substance abuse. After completing KEY, participants may receive transitional treatment at the CREST Outreach Center, a community-based therapeutic community operated in a work-release program (Lockwood & Inciardi, 1993). Evaluation involved follow-ups of graduates of KEY, CREST, and no-treatment inmates who participated in a separate work-release program. At 18-month follow-up, 29% of clients who participated in both KEY and CREST were rearrested, compared with 52% of those in the KEY prison TC program only and 70% of the comparison group (Inciardi et al., 1997).

Evaluations of the Forever Free treatment program at the California Institution for Women have also supported the importance of continuing care in the community. In one study (Jarman, 1993), 90% of prison program graduates who entered and remained in community-based treatment for 5 months or more had a successful parole outcome (i.e., discharged from parole with no return to custody), compared with 72% of graduates who entered community-based treatment but dropped out early, 62% of graduates with no community treatment, and 38% of in-prison program dropouts. A second evaluation of this program (Prendergast, Wellisch, & Wong, 1996) confirmed the benefits of continuing treatment in the community, finding that over two-thirds of Forever Free graduates who entered residential treatment were successful on parole, compared with about one-half of program graduates who did not enter residential treatment and one-fourth of inmates who did not receive treatment in prison.

Finally, a recent evaluation of prison-based treatment within the Federal Bureau of Prisons, which used a quasi-experimental design, paid particular attention to the issue of selection bias (Pelissier et al., 1998; Pelissier et al., in press). The study included men and women who received residential treatment at 20 in-prison treatment programs, and employed two comparison groups, one made up of prisoners in facilities where treatment was unavailable and a second made up of prisoners who were housed at an institution with substance abuse treatment but who did not volunteer for treatment. After controlling for individual- and system-level selection bias, the authors found significant reductions in post-treatment drug use and arrests at six months post-release. In addition, their selection-bias analysis revealed that inmates who were *more* likely to be arrested or to use drugs post-release were selected into the treatment programs. Therefore, if the authors had not controlled for selection bias, the effects of treatment would have been reduced (Pelissier et al., 1998; Pelissier, in press; for three year outcomes, see Pelissier et al., 2000).

MULTIPLE OUTCOMES

Table 1 summarizes the outcome measures reported in the studies of prison-based treatment mentioned above. In all of the studies, the published findings focus on one or two dichotomous outcome variables related to recidivism, generally rearrest and/or reincarceration. Drug use is sometimes included as an outcome variable. For most of these studies, more specific and varied outcome data were collected, but so far, the researchers have not published them. The focus on recidivism in published studies is understandable since rearrest or reincarceration are usually based on official records and thus avoid the bias in self-reporting. It should be noted, however, that records have their own biases and limitations, and, as Knight, Hiller, and Simpson (1999) observe, even with common outcome variables, detailed comparisons of relapse and recidivism rates across these evaluations are complicated by variations in measurement of outcomes. In addition, for correctional systems that fund prison-based treatment programs, recidivism (usually reincarceration) is the outcome of greatest interest. Other outcomes, such as employment and psychological improvement, may have social value, but they are of secondary interest to funding decisions for prison treatment programs. The impact of treatment on drug use is intrinsically relevant to the objective of treatment programs, but an interest in drug use outcomes within the criminal justice system also follows from the close association between drug use and crime. Prison-based treatment programs are premised on the assumption that reductions in drug use as a result of treatment will result in reductions in crime following release.

Considering only rearrest or reincarceration, however, conceals the behavior of treatment and comparison subjects that lead to their return to correctional supervision. How long do offenders remain in the community until rearrest? What crimes do they commit? What are the reasons for return (parole violation, new term)? How serious is the commitment offense? How long do they spend incarcerated? An examination of the effectiveness of prison-based treatment programs using a range of outcome types, measures, and analytic

☐ *Table 1: Outcome Measures Reported in Evaluations of Prison-Based Therapeutic Community Programs*

Treatment Program	Outcome Variable	Source of Outcome Data
Stay'n Out[1]	Rearrest	
	Time until rearrest	Official records
	Successful parole discharge	
Cornerstone[2]	Rearrest	
	Conviction	Official records
	Reincarceration	
KEY/CREST[3]	Rearrest	Follow-up interviews: Self-report
	Drug use	Blood and urine testing
New Vision[4]	Reincarceration	Official records
Amity/R. J. Donovan[5]	Reincarceration	Official records
	Days until reincarceration	
Forever Free[6]	Reincarceration	Official records
	Successful parole discharge	
TRIAD[7]	Rearrest	Official records
	Drug use	Probation officer reports

[1]Wexler, Falkin, & Lipton (1990)
[2]Field (1985, 1992)
[3]Martin, Butzin, Saum, & Inciardi (1999)
[4]Knight, Simpson, & Hiller (1999)
[5]Wexler, Melnick, Lowe, & Peters (1999)
[6]Prendergast, Wellisch, & Wong (1996)
[7]Pelissier et al. (In press)

methods would provide a more complete understanding of the impact of these programs and addresses the interests of a broader audience than correctional officials. In particular, economic analyses of prison-based treatment that include local criminal justice processing costs would benefit from information about number of arrests, types of charges, and case dispositions, in addition to return-to-custody rates.

The purpose of this paper is to examine the impact of the Amity prison treatment program at 12 months following release to parole using multiple measures of outcomes related to crime and drug use. Where appropriate, survival analysis is used to compare differences in time to event among the study groups.

AMITY TREATMENT PROGRAM AND EVALUATION

Program Description

The Amity prison TC was established as a demonstration project funded by the California Department of Corrections in 1990. The Amity TC is located at the R. J. Donovan Correctional Facility, a medium-security prison near San Diego (the program is described in more detail in Graham & Wexler, 1997; Wexler, De Leon, Thomas, Kressel, & Peters, 1999; Wexler, Melnick, Lowe, & Peters, 1999; Winnet, Lowe, Mullen, & Missakian, 1992). The program provides intensive treatment to 200 male inmates who reside in a dedicated housing unit during the last 9 to 12 months of their prison term. All participants volunteer for the program. Formal programming occurs four hours a day during the week (with the other four hours being devoted to work assignment), but the presence of specially trained and supervised "lifers" who serve as live-in staff ensures that the TC culture and environment is supported 24 hours a day.

As is typical of many TC programs, Amity uses a three-phase treatment model. The first phase of treatment (2-3 months duration) involves clinical observation and assessment of resident needs and problem areas and begins the assimilation process into the TC culture. Orientation to the prison TC procedures and activities occurs through encounter groups, peer structure, and other TC basics. During the second phase (5-6 months duration), residents earn positions of increased responsibility through program involvement and hard emotional work. Education, encounter groups, and counseling sessions focus on self-discipline, self-worth, self-awareness, respect for authority, and acceptance of guidance for problem areas. During the third phase (1-3 months duration), inmates prepare for community re-entry, strengthen their skills in planning and decision making, and design post-discharge plans with guidance from treatment and parole staff.

Upon release from prison, program graduates may volunteer to participate in residential treatment for 6-12 months at an Amity-operated facility called Vista, which houses up to 40 residents at a time. The program content and activities continues and builds upon the prison TC curriculum and is individualized based on the progress achieved in the prison treatment program. Under staff supervision, residents have responsibility for security, facility maintenance, and members' emotional health. All Amity graduates are also encouraged to participate in self-help groups (e.g., AA, NA) and other community services as needed. Amity also operates a drop-in center for program graduates that provides counseling and evening groups to encourage recovery and provide peer support.

Amity Evaluation Design and Sample

Under a NIDA-funded grant to the Center for Therapeutic Community Research at National Development and Research Institutes, Inc., Wexler conducted a prospective 12-month outcome study of the Amity program using a treatment-control group design with random assignment. An eligible pool was created from a waiting list of volunteers who met the prison TC admission criteria. As bed space became available, inmates in the eligible pool were randomly selected and assigned to the treatment condition. The random assignment procedure stratified for approximately equal ethnic proportions. Inmates who were not selected into treatment remained in the eligible pool until they had less than nine months to serve on their prison term, at which point they were removed from the eligible pool and became members of the control group. The final sample consisted of 425 subjects in the treatment group and 290 in the no-treatment group. Data were collected on inmates upon admission to the Amity program or selection into the control group, during the prison TC treatment and community TC aftercare program (for treatment participants only), and at 12 months after release from prison. Criminal justice records data were collected on all 715 subjects, but in part because of funding limitations, 18% of the intake sample was deemed not eligible for the 12-month interview: 9.7% had less than 12 months in the community at the time the follow-up interviews were being conducted, 7.3% lived more than 150 miles from the research site, and 1.0% had special conditions attached to their parole (e.g., Immigration and Naturalization Service holds for deportation). Thus, 587 subjects (82%) were eligible for a 12-month follow-up interview. Of those eligible, 3.2% could not be located, 3.2% refused to participate, and 1.4% had died, resulting in a follow-up interview rate of 90% of the subjects eligible for follow-up (N = 531) or 74% of the original sample (335 in the intent-to-treat group and 196 in the control group).

Table 2 shows characteristics of the full sample and the treatment and the control groups. Of the demographic and background variables examined, the groups differed significantly only on education, with the control group reporting a slightly higher level of educational attainment than the treatment group. For the sample as a whole, the average age was 31, and the ethnic distribution was 38% white, 22% Latino, and 30% African American. Additionally, most had relatively low levels of education and had been employed as non-skilled laborers who earned most of their income from illegal activities. Most had children, but few lived with them prior to arrest and confinement. Subjects reported many childhood problems: 39% had been either physically or sexually abused, 53% had run away from home, and 90% had behavior problems in school. Psychological disturbance was common: 68% had experienced serious depression, 61% had experienced serious anxiety, 46% reported trouble controlling violent behavior, 11% had attempted suicide, and 59% had received some type of psychological treatment. Study participants were primarily users of stimulants and injected drugs. They were at high risk for HIV infection, with 58% being injection drug users and 43% reporting having used shared needles for an overall average of 30 times. Most subjects had a history of violence, with 75% reporting that they had committed either assault, kidnapping, rape,

☐ **Table 2: Comparison of Participants in the TC Intent-to-Treat Group and the Control Group on Selected Background Characteristics**

Variable	Label	Total Sample (n = 715) %	Intent-to-Treat Group (n = 425) %	Control Group (n = 290) %	Comparison of Study Groups p Value*
Age	Mean	30.9	31.2	30.5	n.s.
Ethnicity	Caucasian	37.8	39.5	35.3	n.s.
	African-American	30.1	28.4	32.5	
	Hispanic	22.4	22.9	21.6	
	Other	9.7	9.2	10.6	
Education	< HS Diploma	42.2	42.8	41.4	.03
	HS Diploma Only	53.0	54.1	51.4	
	> HS Diploma	4.8	3.0	7.2	
Marital Status	Married/Living with Partner	39.2	37.6	41.4	n.s.
	Separated/Divorced/ Widowed	20.6	21.3	19.9	
	Never Married	40.3	41.1	38.7	
Employment	Last Twelve Months	34.5	34.0	35.3	n.s.
Criminality in Lifetime	Arrested: Before Age 18	73.8	75.1	72.0	n.s.
	Arrested: Violence Against Persons	55.4	57.0	53.1	n.s.
	Arrested: Weapons Offenses	49.0	47.3	51.4	n.s.
	Arrested: Drugs Sales	49.0	49.6	47.9	n.s.
	Arrested: Drug Possession	79.6	80.6	78.1	n.s.
AIDS Risk in Lifetime	Injected Drugs	57.6	59.1	55.0	n.s.
	Injected with Dirty Needles	62.8	64.3	60.5	n.s.
	Used Needles with Stranger	25.2	24.7	26.5	n.s.
	Engaged in Unprotected Sex	97.1	96.2	98.3	n.s.
Psychiatric Diagnoses	Anti-Social Personality Disorder	51.5	51.6	51.3	n.s.
	Phobias	17.2	17.5	16.8	n.s.
	Post Traumatic Stress Disorder	14.5	14.7	14.0	n.s.
	Depression	10.1	9.2	11.2	n.s.
	Dysthymia	6.9	5.7	8.5	n.s.
	Attention Deficit Hyperactivity Disorder[a]	32.5	33.6	30.5	n.s.

*p value refers to chi square for categorical variables and t-test for continuous variables.
[a] A subsample of 228 subjects completed two ADHD rating scales (146 treatment participants and 82 controls).

or murder. On average, the subjects had been arrested 27 times, had 17 incarcerations, and had spent 6 years in prison.

Amity Outcomes Results

Reincarceration outcomes have been reported for 12- , 24- , and 36-months post-release and are summarized in Figure 1 (Wexler, De Leon, Kressel, & Peters, 1999; Wexler, Melnick, Lowe, & Peters, 1999). At 12-months post-release, statistically significant differences in reincarnation were found for the intent-to-treat and the control subjects (33.9% and 49.7%, respectively). The analysis also examined outcomes among four self-selected subgroups within the treatment group: prison TC dropouts, prison TC completers, aftercare dropouts, and aftercare completers. At 12 months, the reincarceration rate consistently decreased across the four groups, with the aftercare completers showing a reincarceration rate of only 8.2%. At 24 months, the reincarceration rate for all of the groups increased, but the pattern of results was consistent with the 12-month outcomes. The 36-month outcomes continued to show the intent-to-

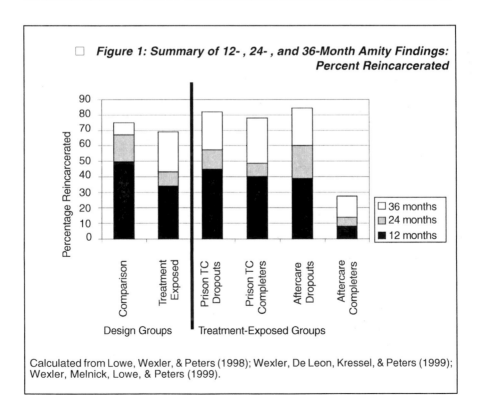

Figure 1: Summary of 12- , 24- , and 36-Month Amity Findings: Percent Reincarcerated

Calculated from Lowe, Wexler, & Peters (1998); Wexler, De Leon, Kressel, & Peters (1999); Wexler, Melnick, Lowe, & Peters (1999).

treatment group with lower reincarceration rates than the control group (69% and 75%, respectively), but the difference was no longer statistically significant. For the inmates who were returned to prison, the published Amity outcome reports also assessed outcomes in terms of the time until reincarceration. Although the data reporting by groups is not consistent across reports, in general, participation in treatment was associated with more days until reincarceration compared with no treatment, as was longer exposure to treatment (Wexler, De Leon, Thomas, Kressel, & Peters, 1999; Wexler, Melnick, Lowe, & Peters, 1999).

STUDY PROCEDURES

The present analysis extends the original 12-month outcome findings by examining a wider range of outcomes, including those based on data from interviews, and using additional analytic techniques, specifically survival analysis. (Although three-year return-to-custody outcomes on the Amity program have been reported [Wexler, Melnick, Lowe, & Peters, 1999], interview data, on which some of the analyses are based, are available only for the 12-month follow-up.) Effect sizes for the main outcomes are also reported. Before presenting the findings, we describe the outcomes variables examined, their source, and the plan of analysis.

Variables

The following outcome variables were included in this analysis:
Crime. Self-report data from the 12-month follow-up interview was used to determine the time (in days) to first illegal activity, type of arrest (at first arrest), and number of months incarcerated (both in jail and prison) during the 12-month follow-up period. Data from the California Department of Corrections provided information on days to first reincarceration and type of reincarceration.
Arrests were grouped into four categories:

> *Drug.* Drinking alcohol, DUI, public consumption/intoxication, use/possession of illegal drug or paraphernalia, sale, distribution, manufacturing of any drug, and forgery of drug prescriptions.

> *Property.* Forgery or fraud, fencing, buying or receiving of stolen property, burglary or auto theft, other theft, larceny, shoplifting, and vandalism.

Violent. Robbery, armed robbery, mugging, rape, murder, violence against other persons, aggravated assault, kidnapping, threatening with a weapon, and arson.

Other. Gambling, running numbers, bookmaking, prostitution or pimping, weapons offenses, vagrancy, loitering, trafficking people across the border, and all others.

Reincarcerations are of three types:

Drug return. Parole agents may return a parolee who is using drugs to a special treatment unit in prison for a limited time (usually 30 days).

Parole violation. Parolees who violate the conditions of parole may be sent back to prison, for an average of about 5 months (CDC, 2000d).

New term. Parolees who are convicted of a new crime receive a new sentence appropriate to the crime, usually for a longer period than for a parole violation.

Drug use. Time to first drug use was calculated from subjects' self-reports. Hair or nail samples were obtained from all subjects not in custody (subjects provided samples voluntarily, refusal rate was 8%) and were analyzed using gas chromatography/mass spectrometry.

Analysis Plan

The analyses examine outcomes between all subjects in the treatment group and the control group for whom follow-up data were available. This "intent-to-treat" analysis is the most conservative test of treatment effectiveness. In addition, following the approach used in previous reports on the Amity study (Wexler, DeLeon et al., 1999; Wexler, Melnick et al., 1999), we have broken out the results for the treatment subjects into four groups by amount of treatment exposure: in-prison TC dropouts, in-prison TC completers, aftercare dropouts, and aftercare completers.

On the basis of previous findings from the Amity and other prison treatment programs, it was expected that the Amity treatment group would have significantly better outcomes than the control group and that, within the treatment group, those who received more treatment would have significantly better outcomes than those who received less treatment. Even when statistically significant differences among the treatment groups were not found, it was expected that the relative outcomes would be ordered in terms of amount of treatment exposure, with the in-prison TC dropouts doing worse and the aftercare completers doing best.

Bivariate comparisons on outcome variables were made between the intent-to-treat group and the control group and among the four treatment-exposed groups. Statistical differences for continuous variables were tested with *t*-tests when comparing the intent-to-treat and the control groups and ANOVA was used when comparing the four treatment groups; chi-square tests were used for categorical variables.

For the variables "days to first illegal activity," "days to first reincarceration," and "days to first drug use," we performed survival analyses using the Kaplan-Meier method. The advantages of this method are that it does not require a normal distribution (the time to the occurrence of an event is usually not normally distributed) and that it allows the inclusion of cases that did not engage in illegal activities or who were not reincarcerated. Scores for subjects reporting no illegal activity or drug use were censored at 365 days. Likewise, reincarceration data was censored at 365 days. These so-called "censored" cases are cases in which the event did not occur during the period of observation. The Kaplan-Meier method creates a survival curve for each group and tests whether the curves are significantly different from one another using the log-rank statistic. All survival analyses were performed using SPSS, version 10.1. As can be seen from the drug use findings that follow, subjects evidently did not include drug use as an illegal activity (i.e., subjects did not report the same amount of time to first drug use as they did for first illegal activity).

For selected 12-month outcomes from the intent-to-treat group and the control group, we calculated effect sizes as the standardized mean difference using the D-STAT program (Johnson, 1993). For means, the effect size is calculated according to the following formula:

$$d = (M_t - M_c)/SD_{pooled}$$

where *d* is the effect size estimate, M_t is the mean of the treatment group, M_c is the mean of the control group, and SD_{pooled} is the pooled standard deviation of the two groups. The D-STAT program (following McNemar, 1962) uses a similar formula for proportions:

$$d = (P_t - P_c)/SD_{pooled}$$

where P_t is the proportion for the treatment group, P_c is the proportion for the control group, and SD_{pooled} is a pooled standard deviation. Reporting effect size is consistent with the increasing use of meta-analysis to synthesize results from multiple studies on a given research topic and with suggestions that researchers supplement statistical significance testing with indexes of treatment magnitude, such as effect size (Cohen, 1994; Wilkinson et al., 1999). Regular reporting of effect sizes in research reports aids in calculations for power analysis and provides estimates of treatment effectiveness needed for cost-benefit and cost-effectiveness analyses.

FINDINGS

Crime

Days to first illegal activity. For subjects' self-reported days to first illegal activity, the Kaplan-Meier survival curves for the intent-to-treat group and the control group were significantly different (Figure 2, logrank $p < .00001$). The mean survival time to the first illegal act was 70.6 days (median 7 days) for the control group and 137.7 days (median 60 days) for the intent-to-treat group. Note that many subjects committed their first illegal act within approximately 60 days following release to parole. Also, by the end of the first year, the large majority of both groups reported committing at least one illegal act. The survival curves for the four treatment-exposed groups showed significant differences (Figure 3, logrank $p < .00001$), with mean survival time for the prison treatment dropouts at 76.2 days (median 10), prison completers at 105.0 days

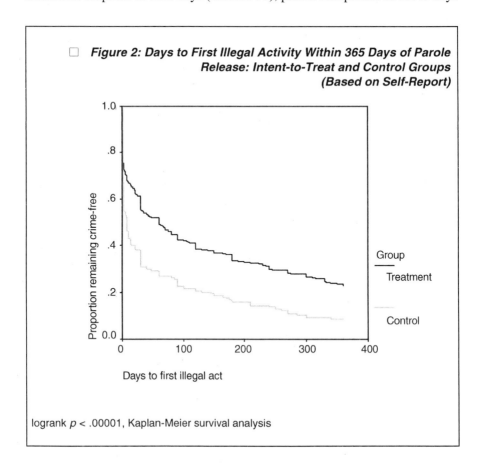

Figure 2: Days to First Illegal Activity Within 365 Days of Parole Release: Intent-to-Treat and Control Groups (Based on Self-Report)

logrank $p < .00001$, Kaplan-Meier survival analysis

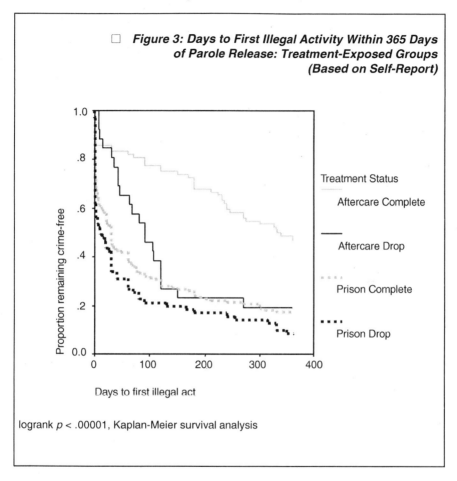

□ **Figure 3: Days to First Illegal Activity Within 365 Days of Parole Release: Treatment-Exposed Groups (Based on Self-Report)**

Treatment Status

Aftercare Complete

Aftercare Drop

Prison Complete

Prison Drop

Days to first illegal act

logrank $p < .00001$, Kaplan-Meier survival analysis

(median 30), aftercare dropouts at 132.3 days (median 90), and aftercare completers at 250.0 days (median 332).

Type of first arrest. Because arrests were not necessarily normally distributed, we used the likelihood ratio chi-square to test for differences between groups. Table 3 presents several comparisons. For all arrests and within each crime category, we compared the intent-to-treat group and the control group and made a separate comparison of the treatment-exposed groups. When we analyzed arrests overall, we found no statistically significant difference between the intent-to-treat group and the control group. Within the treatment-exposed groups, aftercare completers had significantly fewer arrests overall. Within arrest categories, there were no significant differences between the intent-to-treat group and the control group or among the treatment-exposed groups, with the

☐ **Table 3: Type of First Arrest Over 12 Months by Arrest Category and Treatment Status (Based on Self-Report)**

Treatment Status	All Arrests (%)	Arrest Categories (%)		
	Drugs[1]	Property[2]	Violent[3]	Other[4]
Study Groups				
Control (n = 177)	59.9	24.9	18.6	12.4	11.3
Intent-to-Treat (n = 251)	57.4	29.0	12.1	8.1	15.4
Treatment Groups	*		*		
Prison TC Drops (n = 63)	56.3	29.7	9.4	9.5	15.6
Prison TC Completers (n = 123)	64.0	33.3	17.1	8.9	12.8
Aftercare Drops (n = 21)	57.1	23.8	9.5	9.5	23.8
Aftercare Completers (n = 41)	39.0*	17.5	2.5*	2.5	17.1

* $p < .05$, likelihood ratio chi square
[1] Drug arrests include: Drinking alcohol, DUI, public consumption/intoxication, use/possession of illegal drug or paraphernalia, sale, distribution, manufacturing of any drug, and forgery of drug prescriptions.
[2] Property arrests include: Forgery or fraud, fencing, buying or receiving of stolen property, burglary or auto theft, other theft, larceny, shoplifting, and vandalism.
[3] Violent arrests include: Robbery, armed robbery, mugging, rape, murder, violence against other persons, aggravated assault, kidnapping, threatening with a weapon, and arson.
[4] Other arrests include: Gambling, running numbers, bookmaking, prostitution or pimping, weapons offenses, vagrancy, loitering, trafficking people across the border, and all others.

exception of property crimes for which aftercare completers had significantly fewer arrests than did members of the other treatment-exposed groups.

Days to first reincarceration. The Kaplan-Meier survival curves for days to first reincarceration (Figure 4) were significantly different for the control group compared with the intent-to-treat group (logrank $p < .00001$). Mean survival time to first reincarceration was 243 days (median 248) for the control group and 285 days for the intent-to-treat group (median 366, i.e., not reincarcerated). The survival curves for the treatment-exposed groups (Figure 5) were also significantly different (logrank $p < .00001$). Mean time to reincarceration for the prison treatment dropouts was 244 days (median 239), prison completers, 269 days (median 352), aftercare dropouts, 277 days (median 326), and aftercare completers, 352 days (median 366).

Type of reincarceration. For type of reincarceration (Table 4), we compared the control group and the intent-to-treat group and found a significant difference ($p < .01$) between the groups, with a smaller percentage of the in-

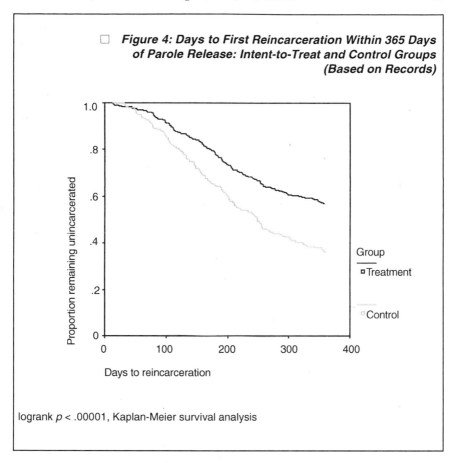

□ **Figure 4: Days to First Reincarceration Within 365 Days of Parole Release: Intent-to-Treat and Control Groups (Based on Records)**

logrank *p* < .00001, Kaplan-Meier survival analysis

tent-to-treat group reincarcerated for new charges and parole violations, a slightly larger percentage reincarcerated in the drug/limited return category, and a larger percent not reincarcerated. Next, we compared the treatment-exposed groups and found significant differences (*p* < .01) among the groups. Higher percentages of those who dropped out of prison treatment were reincarcerated and for more serious violations (e.g., parole violations and new charges rather than for drug/limited return). Also, aftercare completers had dramatically lower percentages in all reincarceration categories.

Mean months incarcerated. Over the 12 months of the follow-up period, the intent-to-treat group had a significantly lower mean number of months incarcerated relative to the control group (Table 5, independent samples *t*-test, *p* < .001). Subjects in the control group spent an average of 4.7 months in prison compared with 3.0 months for the intent-to-treat group. Table 5 also shows

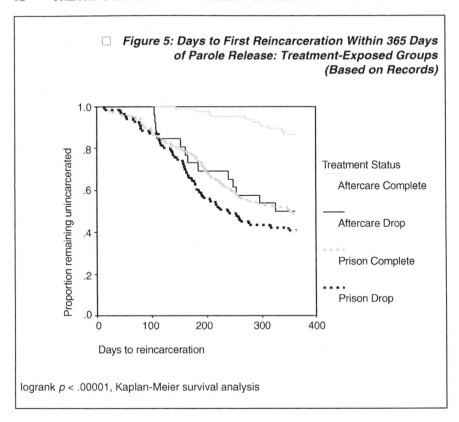

☐ **Figure 5: Days to First Reincarceration Within 365 Days of Parole Release: Treatment-Exposed Groups (Based on Records)**

logrank $p < .00001$, Kaplan-Meier survival analysis

that the aftercare completers had significantly fewer months incarcerated when compared with the other treatment-exposed groups (ANOVA, $p < .001$).

Drug Use

Time to first use. The Kaplan-Meier survival curves for time to first self-reported drug use were significantly different for the intent-to-treat group and the control group (Figure 6, logrank $p < .00001$) and for the treatment-exposed groups (Figure 7, logrank $p < .00001$). The control group had a mean of 31 days to first drug use (median 1), while the intent-to-treat group had a mean of 77 days (median 15). Among the treatment-exposed groups, the prison treatment dropout group had a mean of 32 days to first drug use (median 1), the prison completers, 62 days (median 7), the aftercare dropouts, 91 days (median 45), and the aftercare completers, 184 days (median 180).

Drug test results. Combined results of hair and nail tests obtained at 12-month follow-up showed no significant difference between the intent-to-treat

Table 4: Type of Reincarceration Over 12 Months by Treatment Status (Based on Official Records)

Treatment Status	Not Returned		Drug/ Limited Return[1]		Parole Violation		New Charge	
	N	%	N	%	N	%	N	%
Study Groups (N = 526)**								
Control	44	22.6	17	8.7	76	39.0	58	29.7
Intent-to-Treat	135	40.8	35	10.6	85	25.7	76	23.0
Treatment Groups (N = 331)**								
Prison TC Drops	16	22.5	6	8.5	26	36.6	23	32.4
Prison TC Completers	45	30.0	19	12.7	44	29.3	42	28.0
Aftercare Drops	10	38.5	4	15.4	7	26.9	5	19.2
Aftercare Completers	64	76.2	6	7.1	8	9.5	6	7.1

** $p < .01$ likelihood ratio chi square
[1] Returns for 30-90 days for positive or missed drug test. Returnees in this category are usually enrolled in additional drug treatment during this period of reincarceration.

Table 5: Mean Months Incarcerated in the Year Following Release to Parole by Treatment Status (Based on Self-Report)

Treatment Status	Months Incarcerated Mean (SD)
Study Groups*	
Control (n = 195)	4.71 (3.92)
Intent-to-treat (n = 331)	3.03 (3.70)
Treatment Groups**	
Prison TC Drops (n = 71)	4.49 (3.95)
Prison TC Completers (n = 150)	3.67 (3.68)
Aftercare Drops (n = 26)	2.69 (3.18)
Aftercare Completers (n = 84)	0.76 (2.47)

* $p < .001$, t-test, unequal variances assumed
** $p < .001$, ANOVA

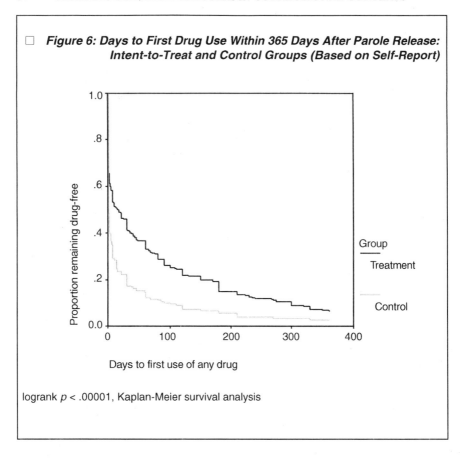

☐ **Figure 6: Days to First Drug Use Within 365 Days After Parole Release:
Intent-to-Treat and Control Groups (Based on Self-Report)**

logrank $p < .00001$, Kaplan-Meier survival analysis

and the control groups. Among the treatment-exposed groups, aftercare completers had significantly fewer positive test results than the other treatment-exposed groups (Table 6).

Effect Sizes

Effect sizes and 95% confidence intervals for selected outcome comparisons between the intent-to-treat group and the control group are shown in Table 7. Effect sizes with a positive sign indicate that the treatment group had a more favorable outcome than the control group. If the confidence interval range includes zero, the effect size is not statistically different from 0.0. In terms of assessing the statistical significance of differences between groups, the results reported in Table 7 are consistent with those reported in the other tables, but the effect sizes supplement statistical significance testing by quanti-

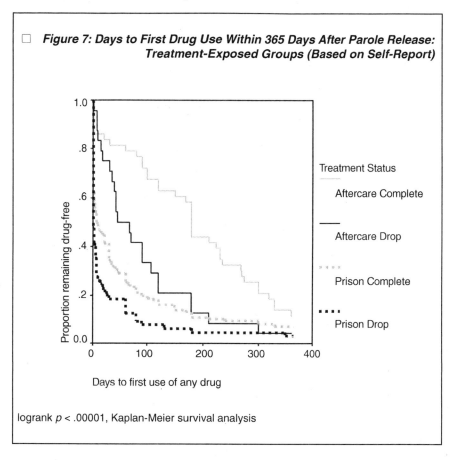

Figure 7: Days to First Drug Use Within 365 Days After Parole Release: Treatment-Exposed Groups (Based on Self-Report)

logrank *p* < .00001, Kaplan-Meier survival analysis

fying the magnitude of the outcome difference between the treatment group and the control group.

DISCUSSION AND LIMITATIONS

Findings from this analysis of multiple outcomes from a 12-month follow-up study of the Amity prison treatment program show that the prisoners who were assigned to treatment performed significantly better on most of the measures examined than those who were assigned to the control group. Notably, days to first illegal activity, days to first incarceration, and days to first use were significantly delayed for the intent-to-treat group. The two groups also significantly differed on the type of reincarceration and the mean number of months incarcerated. Not all measures revealed statistically significant differ-

☐ **Table 6: Subjects Testing Positive for Illicit Drugs at 12-Month Follow-Up by Treatment Status**

Treatment Status	Percent Positive
Study Groups	
Control (n = 59)	61.0
Intent-to-treat (n = 170)	52.9
Treatment Groups***	
Prison TC Drops (n = 25)	76.0
Prison TC Completers (n = 66)	63.6
Aftercare Drops (n = 13)	53.8
Aftercare Completers (n = 66)	33.3

*** $p < .0001$, likelihood ratio chi square

☐ **Table 7: Effect Sizes (as Standardized Mean Differences) and Confidence Intervals for Outcome Measures: Intent-to-Treat and Control Groups**

Outcome Variable	Effect Size	95% CI
Arrest[1]	0.05	−0.14, +0.24
Reincarceration[2]	0.39	+0.21, +0.57
Mean Months Incarcerated[3]	0.44	+0.26, +0.62
Positive Drug Test[4]	0.16	−0.13, +0.46

Note: CI = Confidence Interval
[1]See Table 3
[2]See Table 4
[3]See Table 5
[4]See Table 6

ences between the two groups, however, even though the direction of effect favored the treatment over the control group. We found no differences in type of first arrest and drug test results. The findings indicate that subjects who completed both prison-based treatment and community-based treatment performed significantly better than did those subjects who received lesser amounts of treatment on every measure.

Typical reporting of recidivism data consists of a dichotomous variable represented by the percentage of subjects who have been rearrested or reincarcerated. This ignores the fact that the length of time to a parolee's rearrest or reincarceration has implications for programming and for costs. An outcome evaluation of a prison-based treatment program may have found that the treatment group and the no-treatment group had similar (nonsignificant) levels of returns to custody, but the average time to return for the treatment group was twice as long as that of the no-treatment group, which has cost implications for law enforcement, the courts, and the prison system. Such time-to-event information is captured through survival curves. In our analysis, the survival curves show that aftercare dropouts initially performed better than the prison completers did, but by four to six months after release, the curves overlap. This suggests that participation in community residential treatment keeps parolees out of trouble so long as they remain in treatment, but their dropping of treatment before receiving the planned "dose" tends to lead to relapse or recidivism at rates equivalent to those who received prison treatment only. The treatment implications of this finding require further research, but it would not be evident using a simple dichotomous recidivism variable.

Several limitations in the present study could affect the validity or generalizability of the findings. First, although treatment and control group assignment was random, the treatment groups (prison dropouts, prison completers, aftercare dropouts, aftercare completers) were the result of self-selection. Self-selection bias was controlled in the prison phase of the study through random assignment; but, because participation in aftercare was voluntary, self-selection was not controlled in the aftercare phase. The degree to which self-selection contributed to the better performance of the aftercare completers would require further analysis. One interpretation would be that treatment serves to filter out the less motivated and/or the more dysfunctional participants, leaving only "successes"–those who are highly motivated and have adequate personal and social resources–among those who complete treatment. Thus, the better outcomes for the aftercare completer group may be due, at least partially, to client characteristics rather than to the impact of treatment alone. Sorting out the differential contributions to outcomes of treatment and client characteristics (or other non-treatment factors) is a task of future research.

Second, time spent in local jails is not reflected in the incarceration data obtained from the California Department of Corrections; however, self-report data on the time spent incarcerated does include jail time.

Third, because the interview staff was not able to collect hair and nail samples from incarcerated subjects and because not all of the remaining interviewed subjects agreed to provide hair or nail samples, the number of samples was reduced and the results are possibly biased in a unknown way. The most that can be said regarding the drug test results is that of those subjects who were interviewed in the community and who provided samples for analysis, those who had completed both in-prison and community treatment were significantly less likely than those in the other treatment groups to have used drugs recently.

CONCLUSIONS

Although the overall results from this analysis support the effectiveness of prison-based treatment, it is also clear that, in this study at least, conclusions about the effectiveness of a treatment program may vary depending on which outcomes were selected. Focusing on only one or two outcomes may mask the impact of treatment on other outcome domains that are of interest to various stakeholders. Using a wider range of outcomes from prison-based TC treatments programs than is typically the case provides a more complete and nuanced understanding of the impact of treatment on crime and drug use. It is understandable that those who fund and operate correctional treatment programs would be most interested in whether inmates who receive treatment in prison are less likely to return to custody than those who do not. Beyond the effectiveness of prison-based treatment are cost issues, namely, whether funds devoted to treatment produce cost savings. Answers to both questions rely primarily on percentage returned to custody over a given period of time, some type of comparison condition, and data on various types of costs.

This focus on the dichotomous outcome of return to custody, however, simplifies a more complex story about the impact of treatment. Even if treated inmates did return to prison in the same proportion as non-treated inmates, it would be important to know whether the treatment group recidivists stayed out of prison longer than the non-treatment recidivists and whether the type of return—and, therefore, the amount of time spent back in prison—differed between the two groups. A parole violation does not usually involve the commission of a crime and results in a shorter term than a new charge. In addition, the impact of prison treatment programs extends beyond the state correctional system to local jurisdictions and to society generally. A reduction in drug use and associated criminal activities translates into improved public safety and in fewer arrests, trials, and jail commitments. Again, the typical focus of prison-treatment evaluations on reincarceration masks the broad benefits of such treatment outside of the context of correctional systems.

The results of the survival analysis suggest that the most vulnerable time for relapse or recidivism, whether or not the person has received treatment in prison, is in the month or two just after release to parole. This finding highlights the importance of providing the opportunity for parolees with histories of drug problems to enter community-based treatment, possibly as a condition of parole, and of the need for treatment programs to teach or reinforce relapse prevention techniques with parolees. It also speaks to the importance of assisting parolees in getting to their assigned community treatment program immediately after their release, rather than letting them return first to their old neighborhood, with its social and behavioral reinforcements for drug use and crime.

The findings from this analysis of the Amity treatment program support the argument that prison-based treatment programs (particularly when followed by treatment in the community) are effective, and these results are consistent with other evaluations of such programs. The situation is more complex since treated prisoners did better than non-treated prisoners on some, but not all, of the outcomes examined. No one of the outcome measures examined is clearly privileged in determining the effectiveness of prison-based treatment; stakeholders, depending on their societal perspective, are likely to be interested in or find useful some outcomes and not others and would assess effectiveness accordingly. Although there are limits to the number of outcomes (or types of outcomes) that an evaluator can report, the results of this study would seem to argue for including more rather than fewer outcomes in assessing the impact of prison-based substance abuse treatment.

REFERENCES

Anglin, M. D., Danila, B., Ryan, T., & Mantius, K. (1996). *Staying in Touch: A Fieldwork Manual of Tracking and Procedures for Locating Substance Abusers for Follow-up Studies.* Washington, DC: Center for Substance Abuse Treatment, National Evaluation and Technical Assistance Center.

Anglin, M. D., Longshore, D., & Turner, S. (1999). Treatment alternatives to street crime: An evaluation of five programs. *Criminal Justice and Behavior, 26*(2), 168-195.

Anglin, M. D., Longshore, D., Turner, S., McBride, D., Inciardi, J., & Prendergast, M. (1996). *Studies of the Functioning and Effectiveness of Treatment Alternatives to Street Crime (TASC) Programs* [Final report]. Los Angeles: UCLA Drug Abuse Research Center.

Anglin, M. D., & Perrochet, B. (1998). Drug use and crime: A historical review of research conducted by the UCLA Drug Abuse Research Center. *Substance Use and Misuse, 33*(9), 1871-1914.

Ball, J. C., Rosen, L., Flueck, J. A., & Nurco, D. N. (1981). The criminality of heroin addicts: When addicted and when off opiates. In J. A. Inciardi (Ed.), *The Drugs-Crime Connection* (pp. 39-65). Beverly Hills: Sage Publications.

Burdon, W. M. (1999). Help-seeking behaviors among released male inmates with HIV/AIDS: A test of a proposed theoretical model. Unpublished doctoral dissertation, Claremont Graduate University, Claremont, CA.

Bureau of Justice Statistics. (1995). *Correctional Populations in the United States–1993* (NCJ-156241). Washington, DC: Bureau of Justice Statistics, U.S. Department of Justice.

Bureau of Justice Statistics. (1999a). Correctional populations in the United States–1996 (NCJ-170013). Washington, DC: Bureau of Justice Statistics, U.S. Department of Justice.

Bureau of Justice Statistics. (1999b). *Prisoners in 1998* (NCJ-175687). Washington, DC: Bureau of Justice Statistics, U.S. Department of Justice.

Bureau of Justice Statistics. (1999c). *Probation and Parole in the United States, 1998* (NCJ-178234). Washington, DC: Bureau of Justice Statistics, U.S. Department of Justice.

Bureau of Justice Statistics. (1999d). *Sourcebook of Criminal Justice Statistics 1999.* Washington, DC: Bureau of Justice Statistics, U.S. Department of Justice.

Bureau of Justice Statistics. (2000). *Correctional Populations in the United States–1997* (NCJ-177613). Washington, DC: Bureau of Justice Statistics, U.S. Department of Justice.

California Department of Corrections. (1998). *California Prisoners and Parolees: 1995 & 1996.* Sacramento: Data Analysis Unit, Offender Information Services Branch, California Department of Corrections.

California Department of Corrections. (2000a). *Characteristics of Population in California State Prisons by Institution, June 30, 2000* [On-line]. Available: www.cdc.state.ca.us/pdf/ichar600.pdf.

California Department of Corrections. (2000b). *Historical Trends: 1979-1999.* [On-line]. Available: www.cdc.state.ca.us/pdf/hist299.pdf.

California Department of Corrections. (2000c). *Characteristics of the California Felon Parolees Supervised by the California Department of Corrections, December 31, 1999.* [On-line]. Available: www.cdc.state.ca.us/pdf/pchar99.pdf.

California Department of Corrections. (2000d). California prisoners and parolees, 2000. Sacramento: Data Analysis Unit, Offender Information Services Branch, California Department of Corrections.

Camp, C. G., & Camp, G. M. (1998). *The Corrections Yearbook 1998.* Middletown, CT: Criminal Justice Institute, Inc.

Center for Substance Abuse Treatment. (1998). *Continuity of Offender Treatment for Substance Use Disorders from Institution to Community* (Treatment Improvement Protocol (TIP) Series 30). Washington, DC: Substance Abuse and Mental Health Services Administration, Department of Health and Human Services.

Chaiken, M. R. (1986). Crime rates and substance abuse among types of offenders. In B. D. Johnson & E. Wish (Eds.), *Crime Rates Among Drug-Abusing Offenders.* Final Report to the National Institute of Justice. New York: Narcotic and Drug Research, Inc.

Chaiken, J. M., & Chaiken, M. R. (1990). Drugs and predatory crime. In M. Tonry & J. Q. Wilson (Eds.), *Drugs and Crime* (pp. 203-239). Chicago: University of Chicago Press.

Cohen, J. (1988). *Statistical Power Analysis for the Behavioral Sciences* (2nd ed.). Hillsdale, NJ: L. Erlbaum Associates.

Cohen, J. (1994). The earth is round (p < .05). *American Psychologist, 49,* 997-1003.

Collins, J. J., Hubbard, R. L., Rachel, J. V. Cavanaugh, E. R., & Craddack, S. G. (1982). *Criminal Justice Clients In Drug Treatment.* Research Triangle Park, NC: Research Triangle Institute.

Deitch, D., Koutsenok, I., & Ruiz, A. (2000). The relationship between crime and drugs: What we have learned in recent decades. *Journal of Psychoactive Drugs, 32*(4), 391-397.

Drug Courts Program Office. (1997). *Defining Drug Courts: The Key Components.* Washington, DC: Office of Justice Programs, U.S. Department of Justice.

Duncan, S., Gossop, M., Marsden, J., & Rolfe, A. (2000). Drug misuse and acquisitive crime among clients recruited to the National Treatment Outcomes Research Study. *Criminal Behaviour & Mental Health, 10*(1), 10-20.

Field, G. (1985). The Cornerstone program: A client outcome study. *Federal Probation, 49,* 50-55.

Field, G. (1992). Oregon prison drug treatment programs. In C. G. Leukefeld & F. M. Tims (Eds.), *Drug Abuse Treatment in Prisons and Jails* (Nida Research Monograph Series 118, Pp. 142-155). Rockville, MD: National Institute On Drug Abuse.

Goldkamp, J. S. (1994). *Justice and Treatment Innovation: The Drug Court Movement.* Washington, DC: Office of Justice Programs, U.S. Department of Justice.

Hubbard, R. L., Collins, J. J., Rachel, J. V., & Cavanaugh, E. R. (1988). The criminal justice client in drug abuse treatment. In C. G. Leukefeld & F. M. Tims (Eds.), *Compulsory Treatment of Drug Abuse: Research and Clinical Practice* (NIDA Research Monograph 86, pp. 57-80). Rockville, MD: National Institute on Drug Abuse.

Inciardi, J. A., Martin, S. S., Butzin, C. A., Hooper, R. M., & Harrison, L. D. (1997). An effective model of prison-based treatment for drug-involved offenders. *Journal of Drug Issues, 27*(2), 261-278.

Inciardi, J. A., McBride, D. C., & Rivers, J. E. (1996). *Drug Control and the Courts.* Thousand Oaks, CA: Sage.

Jarman, E. (1993). *An Evaluation of Program Effectiveness for the Forever Free Substance Abuse Program at the California Institution for Women, Frontera, California.* Report to the Legislature, State of California. Sacramento: Office of Substance Abuse Programs, California Department of Corrections.

Johnson, B. (1993). *DSTAT 1.10: Software for the Meta-analytic Review of Research Literatures.* Hillsdale, NJ: Lawrence Erlbaum Associates, Inc.

Knight, K., Hiller, M. L., & Simpson, D. D. (1999). Evaluating corrections-based treatment for the drug-abusing criminal offender. *Journal of Psychoactive Drugs, 31*(3), 299-304.

Knight, K., Simpson, D. D., Chatham, L. R., & Camacho, L. M. (1997). An assessment of prison-based drug treatment: Texas' in-prison therapeutic community program. *Journal of Offender Rehabilitation, 24*(3/4), 75-100.

Knight, K., Simpson, D. D., & Hiller, M. L. (1999). Three-year reincarceration outcomes for in-prison therapeutic community treatment in Texas. *Prison Journal, 79*(3), 337-351.

Lockwood, D., & Inciardi, J. A. (1993). CREST Outreach Center: A work release iteration of the TC model. In J. A. Inciardi, F. M. Tims, & B. W. Fletcher (Eds.), *Innovative Approaches in the Treatment of Drug Abuse: Program Models and Strategies.* Westport, CT: Greenwood Press.

Lowe, L. (1995). *A Profile of the Young Adult Offender in California Prisons as of December 31, 1989-1994* (Prepared for the Substance Abuse Research Consortium, Spring 1995). Sacramento: Office of Substance Abuse Programs, California Department of Corrections.

Lowe, L., Wexler, H. K., & Peters, J. (1998). *The R. J. Donovan In-prison and Community Substance Abuse Program: Three-Year Return-to-Custody Data.* Sacramento: Office of Substance Abuse Programs, California Department of Corrections.

Martin, S. S., Butzin, C. A., Saum, C. A., & Inciardi, J. A. (1999). Three-year outcomes of therapeutic community treatment for drug-involved offenders in Delaware: From prison to work release to aftercare. *Prison Journal, 79*(3), 294-320.

McBride, D. C., & McCoy, C. B. (1993). The drugs-crime relationship: An analytic framework. *Prison Journal, 73*(3/4), 257-278.

McNemar, Q. (1962). *Psychological Statistics* (3rd ed.). New York: Wiley.

Mumola, C. J. (1999). *Substance Abuse and Treatment, State and Federal Prisoners, 1997: Bureau of Justice Statistics Special Report.* Washington, DC: Office of Justice Programs, U.S. Department of Justice.

Murray, D. W. (1996). Drug abuse treatment in the Federal Bureau of Prisons: A historical review and assessment of contemporary initiatives. In K. E. Early (Ed.), *Drug Treatment Behind Bars: Prison-Based Strategies for Change* (pp. 89-100). Westport, CT: Praeger.

National Center on Addiction and Substance Abuse. (1998). *Behind Bars: Substance Abuse and America's Prison Population.* New York: National Center on Addiction and Substance Abuse at Columbia University.

Office of Applied Studies. (2000). *Substance Abuse Treatment in Adult and Juvenile Correctional Facilities: Findings from the Uniform Facility Data Set 1997 Survey of Correctional Facilities.* Rockville, MD: Office of Applied Studies, Substance Abuse and Mental Health Services Administration.

Office of National Drug Control Policy. (1997). *National Drug Control Strategy.* Washington, DC: White House.

Office of National Drug Control Policy. (1998). *National Drug Control Strategy.* Washington, DC: White House.

Office of National Drug Control Policy. (1999). *National Drug Control Strategy.* Washington, DC: White House.

Ossmann, J. (1999). *Evolution of Continuing Care in California.* Bidder's Conference Presentation. Sacramento, CA: Office of Substance Abuse, California Department of Corrections.

Pacific Southwest Addiction Technology Transfer Center. (1999). *Substance Abuse Services Coordination Agency: Community-Based Organization Handbook.* La Jolla, CA: UCSD Pacific Southwest Addiction Technology Transfer Center.

Pelissier, B., Gaes, G. G., Camp, S. C., Wallace, S. B., O'Neil, J. A., & Saylor, W. G. (1998). *TRIAD Drug Treatment Evaluation Project: Six-Month Interim Report.* Washington, DC: Office of Research and Evaluation, Federal Bureau of Prisons.

Pelissier, B., Rhodes, W., Saylor, W., Gaes, G., Camp, S., Vanyur, S., & Wallace, S. (2000). *TRIAD Drug Treatment Evaluation Project Final Report of Three-Year Outcomes: Part 1.* Washington, DC: Office of Research and Evaluation, Federal Bureau of Prisons.

Pelissier, B., Wallace, S., O'Neil, J. A., Gaes, G. G., Camp, S., Rhodes, W., & Saylor, W. (In press). Federal prison residential drug treatment reduces substance use and arrests after release. *American Journal of Drug and Alcohol Abuse.*

Prendergast, M., Wellisch, J., & Wong, M. (1996). Residential treatment for women parolees following prison drug treatment: Treatment experiences, needs and services, outcomes. *Prison Journal, 76*(3), 253-274.

Speckart, G. R., & Anglin, M. D. (1985). Narcotics and crime: An analysis of existing evidence for a causal relationship. *Behavioral Sciences and the Law, 3*(3), 259-282.

Speckart, G. R. & Anglin, M. D. (1986). Narcotics use and crime: An overview of recent research advances. *Contemporary Drug Problems, 13*, 741-769.

Toborg, M. A., Levin, D. R., Milkman, R. H., & Center, L. J. (1976). *Treatment Alternatives to Street Crimes (TASC) Projects: National Evaluation Program, Phase I Summary Report*. Washington, DC: Government Printing Office.

Tonry, M., & Wilson, J. Q. (Eds.). (1990). *Drugs and Crime*. Chicago: University of Chicago Press.

Wellisch, J., Prendergast, M., & Anglin, M. D. (1993). Criminal justice and drug system linkage: Federal promotion of interagency collaboration in the 1970s. *Contemporary Drug Problems, 20*, 611-650.

Wexler, H. K. (1996a). The Amity prison TC evaluation: Inmate profiles and reincarceration outcomes. Presentation at the California Department of Corrections, Youth and Adult Correctional Agency, Sacramento, November 1996.

Wexler, H. K., Blackmore, J., & Lipton, D. S. (1991). Project REFORM: Developing a drug abuse treatment strategy for corrections. *Journal of Drug Issues, 21*(2), 469-490.

Wexler, H. K., De Leon, G., Kressel, D., & Peters, J. (1999). The amity prison TC evaluation: Reincarceration outcomes. *Criminal Justice and Behavior, 26*(2), 147-167.

Wexler, H. K., Falkin, G. P., & Lipton, D. S. (1990). Outcome evaluation of a prison therapeutic community for substance abuse treatment. *Criminal Justice and Behavior, 17*(1), 71-92.

Wexler, H. K., & Graham, W. F. (1993a). Prison-based therapeutic community for substance abusers: Six-month evaluation findings. Paper presented at the American Psychological Association, Toronto, Ontario.

Wexler, H. K., & Graham, W.F. (1993b). Evaluation of a prison therapeutic community: Relationship between crime and drug histories, psychological profiles, and 6-month outcomes. Paper presented at the American Society of Criminology, Phoenix, AZ, October 1993.

Wexler, H. K., Graham, W.F., Koronkowski, R., & Lowe, L. (1995). *Amity Therapeutic Community Substance Abuse Program Preliminary Return to Custody Data*. New York: Center for Therapeutic Community Research, National Development and Research Institutes, Inc., May 1995.

Wexler, H. K., Melnick, G., Lowe, L., & Peters, J. (1999). Three-year reincarceration outcomes for Amity in-prison therapeutic community and aftercare in California. *Prison Journal, 79*(3), 321-336.

Wilkinson, L., & Task Force on Statistical Inference. (1999). Statistical methods in psychology journals: Guidelines and explanations. *American Psychologist, 54*(8), 594-604.

AUTHORS' NOTES

Michael L. Prendergast, PhD, Director of the Criminal Justice Research Group at the UCLA Integrated Substance Abuse Programs, has been project director or principal investigator of a number of projects funded by the National Institute of Justice to study drug treatment strategies in the criminal justice system. He is currently the principal investigator for the Pacific Coast Research Center of NIDA's Criminal Justice Drug Abuse Treatment Studies. Dr. Prendergast is also involved in several evaluations of treatment programs in correctional settings in California and is the principal investigator of two NIDA-funded studies of treatment within criminal justice settings: a five-year follow-up study of inmates who had participated in an evaluation of the Amity Treatment Program at R. J. Donovan Correctional Facility, and an evaluation of the use of vouchers within a drug court treatment program. He is also a co-principal investigator of the statewide evaluation of California's Substance Abuse and Crime Prevention Act (Proposition 36).

Elizabeth A. Hall, PhD, is a researcher in the UCLA Integrated Substance Abuse Programs' Criminal Justice Research Group. She is currently the principal investigator for "Updating the 'Staying in Touch' Fieldwork Manual" (CSAT), project director for the Pacific Coast Research Center of NIDA's Criminal Justice Drug Abuse Treatment Studies, and for "Therapeutic Community Treatment for Prisoners: Long-Term Outcomes and Costs" (NIDA), and project evaluator for "Evaluating Voucher-Based Contingencies in a Drug Court" (NIDA). She is the author of several reports and papers on aspects of drug treatment effectiveness, drug treatment services, adolescent HIV and pregnancy prevention, qualitative methodology, and program evaluation.

Harry K. Wexler, PhD, is a senior researcher at National Development and Research Institutes (NDRI), where he has directed studies on therapeutic community treatment in prisons, including the landmark studies of the Stay'n Out program in New York and the Amity program in California. Dr. Wexler was the principal investigator of the original evaluation of the Amity treatment program at the R. J. Donovan Correctional Facility. He is currently the principal investigator for the NDRI Colorado Research Center of NIDA's Criminal Justice Drug Abuse Treatment Studies. He is the author of numerous papers on substance abuse treatment in prison, therapeutic community treatment, and HIV prevention for parolees.

Supported by NIDA Grant No. R01DA11483. The authors wish to thank Yan Cao and Babajide Olayinka for their assistance in statistical analysis. They are also grateful to the project interviewers, study participants, Lois Lowe, and Psychemedics for providing them with the study's data. The authors would also like to thank the California Department of Corrections and the Amity Foundation for their assistance during the course of the study.

Address correspondence to Michael L. Prendergast, PhD, UCLA Integrated Substance Abuse Programs, 11050 Santa Monica Blvd., Suite 150, Los Angeles, CA 90025 (E-mail: mlp@ucla.edu).

Treating Substance Abusers in Correctional Contexts: New Understandings, New Modalities. Pp. 95-108.
© 2003 by The Haworth Press, Inc. All rights reserved.
10.1300/J076v37n03_05

Differential Impact of Deterrence vs. Rehabilitation as Drug Interventions on Recidivism After 36 Months

HUNG-EN SUNG

Columbia University

ABSTRACT Deterrence through pain infliction and rehabilitation through therapy and training are often conceptualized as competing practices in crime control. With the resurgence of the diversion movement and therapeutic justice, increasingly more offenders are exposed to a particular combination of incarceration and treatment. Even for offenders diverted into community-based treatment, incarceration remains a central part of their criminal justice experiences. Do incarceration and treatment exercise complementary or conflicting crime reduction effects in drug-addicted offenders who have been both incarcerated and treated? Data from 263 participants of Brooklyn's Drug Treatment Alternative-to-Incarceration program showed that although all subjects were exposed to both incarceration and residential drug treatment, only treatment decreased the likelihood of recidivism. No evidence of deterrence was found, and there were some indications of the criminogenic influence of incarceration among studied subjects. Policy implications are discussed. *[Article copies available for a fee from The Haworth Document Delivery Service: 1-800-HAWORTH. E-mail address: <docdelivery@ haworthpress.com> Website: <http://www.HaworthPress.com> © 2003 by The Haworth Press, Inc. All rights reserved.]*

KEYWORDS Deterrence, rehabilitation, drug offenders, drug treatment, DTAP, diversion, recidivism

Assumptions about addictive behavior lie beneath drug policy-making. Drug policy initiatives are devised, justified, and evaluated based on discernible beliefs about why people use drugs and how society can change the behavior of drug users. Deterrence and rehabilitation are the two traditional penal theories that have fiercely competed in the public and academic arena in regard to explaining and changing drug abuse and other criminal activities.

The concept of deterrence is embedded in the rational-choice analysis of human behavior developed by early classical penologists concerned with judicial reform (Beccaria, 1986; Bentham, 1988). From this perspective, every person is a rational actor involved in end/means calculations and freely chooses law-abiding or law-breaking behaviors based on their rational calculations. All else being constant, choice will be directed towards the maximization of pleasure and the avoidance of pain. Therefore, painful punishments (especially those administered in a swift, severe, certain, and proportional manner) become the key to controlling and decreasing socially harmful behaviors. As result, criminal justice interventions should focus on punishing known deviants in order to prevent them from ever again violating the specific norms they have broken. A good example of deterrent strategies is New York's Rockefeller Drug Laws (enacted in 1973), which impose extremely harsh mandatory sentences on drug offenders. (For example, the possession of four ounces or sale of two ounces of a narcotic substance carries a penalty of 15 years to life in prison.) The concern here is that although motives underneath drug addiction can never be thoroughly delineated for each offender, it is possible to extinguish problematic behavior through the rational use of lengthy imprisonment as a negative sanction.

In contrast, the idea of rehabilitation is rooted in the positivist thinking that promoted widespread scientific advances. Led by 19th century Italian criminologists, positivists are skeptical about deterrence. Instead, their research on the external (social, psychological, and biological) "causes" of crime focused attention on the factors that constrain the rational choice of individual actors (Lombroso, 1918; Ferri, 1899). The positivists prefer to concentrate on reforming and treating the criminal. Proportionality is seen as mistaken, because the criminal is not in control of his criminality, and so fitting punishment to crime will not prevent the commission of further offenses. The theory particularly favors the practice of treatment or rehabilitation. A contemporary application of the philosophy of rehabilitation is the diversion movement that began in 1965-1967 (Walker, 2000). The primary objective of diversion is to get offenders out of the criminogenic environment of jails and prisons and to place them into a therapeutic program where clinical and social services are provided.

While most policy discussions and research studies tend to portray these two intervention approaches as competing schools of thought, the quick advancement of the therapeutic discourse in American criminal justice has made a combination of incarceration and treatment a common experience of offenders with a history of substance abuse. Treatment is now widely available to substance-abusing offenders as either a supplement or an alternative to incarceration. Self-help programs like Narcotics Anonymous have become very common among convicted jail inmates (Wilson, 2000), while one-third of those state and federal prison inmates who used drugs in the month prior to their arrest have been treated for substance abuse or enrolled in other drug abuse programs (Mumola, 1999). It is also estimated that 42% of those probationers who said they were using drugs the month before arrest have received drug treatment during their current sentence (Mumola, 1998). As traditional correctional authorities quickly incorporate treatment into their regular sanctions, innovative diversion programs are created by judges and prosecutors across the country to offer felons and misdemeanants awaiting dispositions opportunities to enter community-based treatment (Inciardi, McBride, & Rivers, 1996; Trone & Young, 1996; Nolan, 2001). For this rapidly growing population of drug-involved offenders who have receive both incarceration (as either pre-trial detention or post-conviction imprisonment) and treatment (as a part of, or a supplement or alternative to their punitive sanctions), deterrence and rehabilitation become complementary interventions to reduce their criminal involvement.

Despite this convergence of incarceration and treatment in current drug crime control, little research attention has focused on this unique phenomenon. Most evaluation studies have adopted a simplistic approach by comparing "treatment" groups with "prison" groups to assess the impact of deterrence and rehabilitation in different subsamples. Yet little is known about how these two competing interventions affect the behavior of offenders who have been exposed to both incarceration and mandated treatment. In the study presented in this paper, I will report results from a study of nonviolent drug-addicted felons who were subjected to both incarceration and treatment during the legal processing of their offenses. Both deterrent and rehabilitative effects on their post-intervention recidivism were measured and compared. These findings contribute to a better understanding of how addictive behavior and related criminal deviance respond to planned governmental interventions.

DETERRENCE AND REHABILITATION AMONG SUBSTANCE-ABUSING OFFENDERS

Theoretically, being arrested and incarcerated and watching others receive the same punishment should inspire respect and fear of criminal justice sanctions among substance abusers and result in less frequent criminal behavior. Nevertheless, empirical support for this policy philosophy is scant. Among different punitive sanctions, only license revocation is associated with declining recidivism among drunk drivers, and incarceration has no significant impact on subsequent infractions (Ross, 1991; Yu, 1994). Findings indicate that rehabilitation efforts appeared to reduce the likelihood of recidivism more than punitive sentences (Taxman & Piquero, 1998). Although perceptions of certain punishment have been found to depress probation violations among participants of intensive drug probation programs (Maxwell & Gray, 2000), successful deterrence among drug offenders through incarceration has not been reported in the United States or anywhere else (Fagan, 1994; Caulkins, Rydell, Schwabe, & Chiesa, 1997; Odegard & Amundsen, 1998). After all, incarceration may not be much more difficult or painful than life outside correctional facilities for offenders from inner-city neighborhoods where prospects for a decent existence are dim. Meanwhile, the prison subculture might actually induce inmates to develop a deeper involvement in the underworld of drugs and crime (Inciardi, McBride, & Rivers, 1996). The deterrent effects of incarceration are questioned for all kinds of offenses and offenders. A recent review of 50 evaluative studies has found that vis-à-vis other alternatives, prison produces slight increases in recidivism, and that low-risk criminals are the most negatively influenced by the incarceration experiences (Gendreau, Goggin, & Cullen, 2000). Based on these results, researchers recommend that offenders not be sentenced to prisons under the expectation that this will reduce their criminal behavior after release.

Treating drug offenders or offenders who commit crime to maintain their drug abuse has a powerful appeal because it is consistent with the public health approach that views addiction as a disease. Supporting evidence for this approach is abundant. Participants of criminal justice-mandated drug treatment programs not only decrease their involvement in criminal activities after treatment (Benedict, Huff-Corzine, & Corzine, 1998), but also show better improvement than their incarcerated counterparts (Eisenberg, 1999; Dynia & Sung, 2000; Peters & Murrin, 2000; Belenko, 2001). Undoubtedly, treatment of drug-addicted offenders will remain an emphasis of American criminal justice policy-making in the first decade of the 21st century (MacKenzie, 1994).

An important weakness in the evaluation design of past studies is the definition of deterrence and rehabilitation as mutually exclusive interventions or experiences. As a standard strategy, researchers routinely contrasted "treatment" offenders with "prison" offenders assuming, at least methodologically, that participants of criminal justice-sponsored treatment were never incarcerated or that prison inmates were never exposed to any significant therapeutic interventions (e.g., Eisenberg, 1999; Dynia & Sung, 2000; Spohn, Piper, Martin, & Frenzel, 2001). This experimental approach ignores the influence of therapeutic jurisprudence in the current administration of justice, which has led to the blurring of the distinction between punishment and treatment, in both theory and practice (Nolan, 2001). There are fewer and fewer pure "prison" or "treatment" substance-abusing offenders under criminal justice supervision nowadays, and more and more hybrid cases that receive both interventions in their criminal justice experiences. The present study addresses this problem by measuring the amount of time that a group of participants in coerced treatment actually spent in both incarceration and treatment, and by analyzing how each of these experiences impacted on their recidivism.

HYPOTHESES

A "middle ground" approach now dominates American drug policy-making, which "includes a general acceptance of current anti-drug policies, but with increased support and funding for drug treatment and prevention" (Belenko, 2000: p. 364). Increasingly more drug-addicted offenders are now exposed to varying doses of incarceration, threat of incarceration, and treatment, during the processing of their cases. To those drug offenders who have been both incarcerated and treated at different stages of their stay in the system, the real issue is how their criminal propensity responds to these two diametrically different strategies. In order to disentangle the impact of each intervention, both deterrence and rehabilitation propositions need to be measured for and tested on the same group of subjects. Hence, I formulate the following hypotheses:

> *Deterrence hypothesis:* The length of incarceration is negatively associated with the likelihood of recidivism.

> *Rehabilitation hypothesis:* The length of treatment is negatively associated with the likelihood of recidivism.

Four different scenarios are plausible. These two hypotheses may be simultaneously corroborated or rejected. If both deterrence and rehabilitation hypotheses are empirically corroborated, incarceration and treatment should compound to maximize crime reduction. It is also possible that only one, either the deterrence hypothesis or the rehabilitation hypothesis, is validated. Any outcome would generate important policy implications.

DATA, VARIABLES, AND ANALYTICAL METHODS

Data for this study were collected from 263 participants of the Drug Treatment Alternative-to-Prison program (DTAP) run by the Kings County (Brooklyn) District Attorney's Office, New York. DTAP diverts prison-bound repeat felony offenders to residential drug treatment. The program targets drug-addicted defendants arrested for nonviolent felony offenses who have previously been convicted of one or more nonviolent felonies. For the first 7 years, DTAP operated as a deferred prosecution program in which the adjudicative process is halted or suspended to allow accepted defendants to participate in residential drug treatment for a period of 15 to 24 months. Those who successfully completed the program had their charges dismissed; those who dropped out or were expelled were brought back to court by a special warrant enforcement team and prosecuted on the original charges. In January 1998, DTAP was shifted from a deferred prosecution program to a deferred sentencing program. Now qualified participants enter a felony guilty plea and receive a deferred sentence that allows them to participate in residential treatment. Those who fail treatment are returned to court and sentenced to prison. All 263 subjects included in this study participated in the old deferred prosecution program.

Official arrest data were examined for the 263 offenders, who were arrested in police undercover operations for drug sales and entered DTAP between December 1990 and December 1992. Of these, 182 successfully completed treatment, and the remaining 81 failed treatment and were subsequently prosecuted and sentenced to prison. Both completers and failures were detained in jail during the pre-admission screening period, which averaged 49.5 days for the entire sample.

Table 1 displays variables used in the analysis. Recidivism was operationally defined as the first official rearrest occurring within the 3-year period following treatment completion or prison release. Therefore, the dependent variable was a dichotomous measure that identified recidivists in the sample. Eighty (30%) of the 263 subjects were rearrested during the 3-year follow-up period. Lengths of incarceration and treatment were the main predictors and reflected the hypothesized conceptual constructs of deterrence and rehabilitation. For those who successfully completed treatment, incarceration time only included the pre-admission detention time, while for those who failed treatment, incarceration time encompassed both the pre-admission detention and the post-treatment imprisonment. Treatment time gauged the period that extended between treatment entry and treatment completion or treatment failure. It is in this sense that all treatment completers and treatment failures experienced both incarceration and treatment.

Following extant literature on correlates of recidivism (Klein & Caggiano, 1986; Gendreau, Little, & Goggin, 1996; Zamble & Quinsey, 1997), I included age, education, employment, and criminal history as control variables in the multivariate analysis, to reduce potential disturbances from factors traditionally associated with recidivism. Among these variables, age and criminal history were of particular importance in that youthfulness and extensive criminal careers regularly surfaced, practically without exception, as the most important predictors of recidivism.

Since the dependent variable is a dichotomous yes/no measure with a latent continuous meaning, Pearson r coefficients and odds ratios from logistic regression analysis were computed (Menard, 1995). The assessment of the statistical and substantive significance of the bivariate correlations, logistic regression coefficients, and odds ratios allowed me to evaluate the empirical plausibility of each of the research hypotheses. Although odds ratios contain the same information as the logistic regression coefficients, they are of more

Table 1: Description of Variables (N = 263)

Name	Description	Rearrested (N = 80)				Not rearrested (N = 183)			
		Mean	SD	#	%	Mean	SD	#	%
Incarceration time	Number of days spent in pre-trial detention and post-sentence incarceration	350.5	355.7	--	--	171.0	256.1	--	--
Treatment time	Number of days spent in residential drug treatment	404.3	292.2	--	--	566.0	227.2	--	--
Age	Number of year at treatment admission	28.2	6.9	--	--	31.0	6.7	--	--
Sex	Male	--	--	66	32.8	--	--	135	67.2
	Female	--	--	14	22.6	--	--	48	77.4
Ethnicity	Black	--	--	20	23.3	--	--	66	76.7
	Hispanic	--	--	55	36.2	--	--	97	63.8
	White	--	--	5	20.0	--	--	20	80.0
Education	Had a high school diploma or GED	--	--	1	4.8	--	--	20	95.2
	Did not have a high school diploma or GED	--	--	64	36.3	--	--	111	63.4
Employment	Worked full-time or part-time	--	--	17	35.4	--	--	31	64.6
	Unemployed	--	--	63	29.3	--	--	152	70.7
Criminal history	Number of prior adult arrests	4.0	4.9	--	--	4.4	5.1	--	--

tangible meaning by conveying changes in the odds of being rearrested. Given the directionality of the hypotheses, one-tailed tests were performed.

FINDINGS

A quick survey of Tables 2 and 3 reveals that consistent with extant research literature (e.g., Klein & Caggiano, 1986; Gendreau, Little, & Goggin, 1996; Zamble & Quinsey, 1997), recidivism among offenders is not easy to predict. Only a few control variables were of relevance for predicting 3-year recidivism in this sample. Among them, age and education exerted the most significant influence on the outcome variable. Those who were rearrested averaged 28 years of age at the time of treatment admission, while the mean age for those who remained crime-free was 31. Only 5% of those who had a high school diploma or a GED were rearrested, as compared to 36% of those who did not have such educational credentials. According to the odds ratios, a one-year increase in age and possession of a high school diploma or a GED decreased the likelihood of being rearrested by 6% and 59%, respectively.

Deterrence Hypothesis

The deterrence hypothesis anticipates a statistically significant negative relationship between the length of incarceration and the likelihood of rearrest. The variable incarceration time was both statistically and substantively significant at the bivariate level, but in the direction opposite that predicted by the deterrence hypothesis. Those subjects who were arrested averaged 351 days in incarceration, while those who did not recidivate spent 171 days in detention. It was evident that treatment dropouts were overrepresented among the group of recidivists (dropouts, 48%; graduates, 23%). This unexpected positive association indicates that the likelihood of being rearrested increased as the offender spent more days in jail or prison.

The counterintuitive bivariate relationship that was statistically significant at 0.0001 level became statistically spurious (logistic regression coefficient = 0.0004) when other factors were held constant in the multivariate logistic model. It suggests that the relationship was heavily contingent on the control variables, especially age and educational attainment. In fact, in treatment retention and recidivism studies using different samples from the DTAP population, age was consistently critical in predicting offenders' behavior during and after treatment (Lang & Belenko, 2000; Dynia & Sung, 2000). According to the observed odds ratio of 1.0004 for incarceration time, a 100-day increase in penal custody resulted in a 4% increase in the odds of being rearrested for this sample. No deterrence effect was found in this sample of 263 drug-addicted felons, and some evidence of the criminogenic influence of incarceration was detected.

☐ **Table 3: Logistic Regression Analysis Predicting 3-Year Recidivism (N = 263)**

Variables	B	SE	Wald Statistic	Odds Ratio
Predicting Variables				
Incarceration time (days)	0.0004	0.0008	0.2928	1.0004
Treatment time (days)	−0.0472*	0.0289*	2.6756*	0.9539*
Control Variables				
Age	−0.0551**	0.0241**	5.2332**	0.9464**
Sex (male)	0.5577	0.3343	2.2613	1.4275
Race/ethnicity (Hispanic)			0.7681	
White	−0.1025	0.3709	0.0549	0.9026
Black	−0.0853	0.4374	0.0866	0.9183
Education	−0.8793***	0.3343***	6.9206***	0.4151***
Employment status	0.2904	0.3694	0.6184	1.3370
Criminal history	0.0076	0.0311	0.0600	1.0077

Note: One-tailed test results are reported.
*p < .05; **p < .01; ***p < .001; ****p < .0001

Rehabilitation Hypothesis

Unlike incarceration time, time spent in residential treatment was statistically and substantively significant at both bivariate and multivariate levels. Subjects who had longer treatment stays were less likely to be rearrested. The average length of treatment was 404 days for the recidivists and 566 days for those who remained crime-free throughout the follow-up period. The moderate negative association between the number of days spent in treatment and the likelihood of recidivating was in the anticipated direction, demonstrating that rehabilitative interventions did have a noticeable impact on DTAP participants' criminal careers.

The Pearson r of −0.2340 and the logistic regression of −0.0472 were statistically significant at the 0.0001 and 0.05 levels, respectively. The odds ratio of 0.9539 revealed that a 100-day increase in treatment length decreased the odds of being rearrested by 461%. Regardless of age and educational background, treatment reduced recidivism. This finding represents a robust backing to the argument that addiction-induced criminal involvement is a treatable disease rather than a rational behavior to be eliminated by inflicting pain to the offender.

□ **Table 2: Correlations for Recidivism and Predictor Variables (N = 263)**

	1	2	3	4	5	6	7	8
Recidivism	-----							
Incarceration time	0.2235****	-----						
Treatment time	-0.2340****	-0.8117****	-----					
Age	-0.1833***	-0.0909	0.0595	-----				
Sex (male)	0.0834	-0.0356	-0.0692	0.0058	-----			
Race (Hispanic)	0.0819	0.0412	-0.0447	-0.0401	0.1721***	-----		
Education	0.1791***	-0.0584	0.0429	0.0951	0.0233	-0.1262*	-----	
Employment	0.0513	-0.0032	-0.0012	-0.0072	0.1697	0.0384	0.0822	-----
Criminal history	-0.394	0.0574	-0.0264	0.2677****	-0.0873	-0.1279*	-0.0058	0.0306

Note: One-tailed test results are reported.
*p < .05; **p < .01; ***p < .001; ****p < .0001

CONCLUSION AND DISCUSSION

Substance-abusing offenders now receive a combination of treatment and incarceration on a regular basis. I tested the deterrence and rehabilitation hypotheses that underlie these criminal justice responses on a sample of 263 DTAP participants. Only one hypothesis prevailed from the analysis. Rehabilitation worked; and only treatment exercised an impact on crime reduction in this sample. Staying in residential drug treatment was of great help to the participants of mandated treatment and effectively created exit opportunities to many career drug offenders. In contrast, incarceration had at best no appreciable effects on recidivism; at worst, jail and prison experiences prolonged the criminal careers of some DTAP participants.

The finding that incarceration is at best an ineffective deterrent weapon in reducing criminal behavior among drug offenders shores up the position of current efforts at reforming draconian mandatory sentence laws for nonviolent drug offenders. Since prison cells could be used to hold more dangerous offenders, the imposition of lengthy prison sentences on nonviolent offenders who have committed crime to support their drug habits is irrational and could be counterproductive. This finding does not imply that drug use needs to be decriminalized, but suggests that we should look for effective solutions beyond locking up addicted offenders. Leaving the public health system to monopolize the issue of drug control will not work neither because the real problem is not only about treatment availability. Making treatment opportunities available to the public is not a sufficient enticement since many drug abusers will enter treatment *only* if coerced. Research has conclusively proved that criminal justice sanctions can enormously increase treatment entry and retention rates as well as positive post-treatment outcomes (National Institute on Drug Abuse, 1999). Rather than abolishing the prohibitions against drugs, the penalties against their use can serve the constructive role of encouraging addicts to opt for treatment.

Integrating criminal justice and drug treatment services could degenerate into an empty slogan if we do not carefully experiment and rigorously evaluate different strategies. Not all mandated treatment models produce success or equal success. For example, the therapeutic community model has been successful in reducing recidivism among prison inmates (Wexler, Falkin, & Lipton, 1990; Inciardi, Martin, Butzin, Hooper, & Harrison 1997); but many prison-based drug treatment programs that did not segregate those in treatment from the general prison population have failed (Gerstein & Harwood, 1990; Knight, Hiller, & Simpson, 1999). More importantly, those who are coerced into community-based treatment by criminal justice authorities often fare as well as, or in some cases even better than, those who enter such programs voluntarily (Hiller, Knight, Broome, & Simpson, 1998; Hynes, 2000). Interpreted vis-à-vis these recent research findings, results from the study presented in this paper argue for an expansion in the criminal justice utilization of community-based residential drug treatment for nonviolent drug users identified by the legal system.

REFERENCES

Beccaria, C. (1986). *On crimes and punishments*. Indianapolis, IN: Hackett.

Belenko, S. R. (2000). "A middle ground?" In S. R. Belenko (Ed.), *Drugs and drug policy in America* (p. 364). Wesport, CT: Greenwood.

Belenko, S. R. (2001). *Research on drug courts: A critical review 2001 update*. New York: The National Center on Addiction and Substance Abuse.

Benedict, W. R., Huff-Corzine, L., & Corzine, J. (1998). "Clean up and go straight": Effects of drug treatment on recidivism among felony probationers. *American Journal of Criminal Justice, 22,*169-187.

Bentham, J. (1988). *A fragment on government*. New York: Cambridge University Press.

Caulkins, J. P., Rydell, C. P., Schwabe, W. L., & Chiesa, J. (1997). *Mandatory minimum drug sentences: Throwing away the key or the taxpayers' money?* Santa Monica, CA: RAND.

Dynia, P. A. & Sung, H. (2000). Safety and effectiveness of diverting felony drug offenders to residential treatment as measured by recidivism. *Criminal Justice Policy Review, 11,* 299-311.

Eisenberg, M. (1999). *Three year recidivism tracking of offenders participating in substance abuse treatment programs*. Rockville, MD: National Institute of Justice.

Fagan, J. A. (1994). Do criminal sanctions deter drug crimes? In D. L. MacKenzie and C. D. Uchida (Eds.), *Drugs and crime: Evaluating public policy initiatives* (pp. 188-214). Thousand Oaks, CA: Sage.

Ferri, E. (1899). *Criminal sociology*. New York: D. Appleton & Co.

Gendreau, P., Little, T., & Goggin, C. (1996). Meta-analysis of the predictors of adult offender recidivism: What works! *Criminology, 34,* 575-607.

Gendreau, P., Goggin, C., & Cullen, F. T. (2000). *Effects of prison sentences on recidivism*. Ottawa: Canada Minister of Public Works and Government Services.

Gerstein, D. R., & Harwood, H. J. (1990). *Treating drug problems*, Vol. 1. Washington, DC: National Academy Press.

Hiller, M. L., Knight, K., Broome, K. M., & Simpson, D. D. (1998). Legal pressure and treatment retention in a national sample of long-term residential programs. *Criminal Justice and Behavior, 25,* 463-481.

Inciardi, J. A., McBride, D. C., & Rivers, J. E. (1996). *Drug control and the courts*. Thousand Oaks, CA: Sage.

Inciardi, J. A., Martin, S. S., Butzin, C. A., Hooper, R. M., & Harrison, L. D. (1997). An effective model of prison-based treatment for drug-involved offenders. *Journal of Drug Issues, 27,* 261-278.

Klein, S. P. & Caggiano, M. N. (1986). *The prevalence, predictability, and policy implications of recidivism*. Santa Monica, CA: RAND.

Knight, K., Hiller, M., & Simpson, D. D. (1999). *Prison-based treatment assessment (PTA): Final activity report*. Rockville, MD: National Institute of Justice.

Lang, M. A., & Belenko, S. R. (2000). Predicting retention in a residential drug treatment alternative to prison program. *Journal of Substance Abuse Treatment, 19,* 145-160.

Lombroso, C. (1918). *Crime: Its causes and remedies*. Boston, MA: Little Brown.

MacKenzie, D. L. (1994). Drug policy initiatives: The next 25 years. In D. L. MacKenzie and C. D. Uchida (Eds.), *Drugs and crime: Evaluating public policy initiatives* (pp. 283-290). Thousand Oaks, CA: Sage.

Maxwell, S. R., & Gray, M. K. (2000). Deterrence: Testing the effects of perceived sanction certainty on probation violations. *Sociological Inquiry, 70*, 117-136.

Menard, S. (1995). *Applied logistic regression.* Thousand Oaks, CA: Sage.

Mumola, C. J. (1999). *Substance abuse and treatment, state and federal prisoners, 1997.* Washington, DC: Bureau of Justice Statistics.

Mumola, C. J. (1998). *Substance abuse and treatment of adults on probation, 1995.* Washington, DC: Bureau of Justice Statistics.

National Institute on Drug Abuse (1999). *Principles of drug addiction treatment: A research-based guide.* Bethesda, MD: National Institute on Drug Abuse.

Nolan, J. L. (2001). *Reinventing justice: The American drug court movement.* Princeton: Princeton University Press.

Odegard, E., & Amundsen, A. (1998). Measuring special deterrence effects on drug offenders. *Studies on crime and crime prevention, 7*, 239-258.

Peters, R. H., & Murrin, M. R. (2000). Effectiveness of treatment-based drug courts in reducing criminal recidivism. *Criminal Justice and Behavior, 27*, 72-96.

Ross, H. L. (1991). License deprivation as a drunk-driver sanction. *Alcohol, Drugs and Driving, 7*, 63-69.

Taxman, F. S., & Piquero, A. (1998). On preventing drunk driving recidivism: An examination of rehabilitation and punishment approaches. *Journal of Criminal Justice, 26*, 129-143.

Trone, J., & Young, D. (1996). *Bridging drug treatment and criminal justice.* New York: Vera Institute of Justice.

Walker, S. (2000). *Sense and nonsense about crime and drugs: A policy guide.* 5th ed. Belmont, CA: Wadsworth.

Wexler, H. K., Falkin, G. P., & Lipton, D. S. (1990). Outcome evaluation of a prison therapeutic community for substance abuse treatment. *Criminal Justice and Behavior, 17*, 71-92.

Wilson, D. J. (2000). *Drug use, testing, and treatment in jails.* Washington, DC: Bureau of Justice Statistics.

Yu, J. (1994). Punishment celerity and severity: Testing a specific deterrence model on drunk driving recidivism. *Journal of Criminal Justice, 22*, 355-366.

Zamble, E., & Quinsey, V. L. (1997). *The criminal recidivism process.* New York: Cambridge University Press.

AUTHOR'S NOTE

Hung-En Sung, PhD, (State University of New York at Albany, 2000), is a research associate at the National Center on Addiction and Substance Abuse at Columbia University (CASA). His research interests revolve around policing, drug abuse, and comparative criminology. Dr. Sung has published a number of journal articles and also a book titled *The Fragmentation of Policing in American Cities: Toward an Ecological Theory of Police-Citizen Relations* (Praeger, 2001).

The author thanks the New York State Division of Criminal Justice Services (DCJS) for permission to use its statewide arrest data and the Kings County District Attorney's Office (KCDA) for permission to access its administrative records. Conclusions and opinions reported in this study are those of the author and do not represent the official position of CASA, DCJS or KCDA.

Address correspondence to Hung-En Sung, PhD, The National Center on Addiction and Substance Abuse at Columbia University, 633 Third Avenue, 19th Floor, New York, NY 10017.

Treating Substance Abusers in Correctional Contexts: New Understandings, New Modalities. Pp. 109-121.
10.1300/J076v37n03_06

Criminal Violence and Drug Use: An Exploratory Study Among Substance Abusers in Residential Treatment

ERIC J. WORKOWSKI

Treatment Trends, Inc.

ABSTRACT This study examined the relationship between criminal violence and type of substance abuse among 184 current and former residents of an inpatient non-hospital drug and alcohol treatment facility. The criminal justice system functioned as the source of referral into the program for 89% of the subjects studied while only 11% came to treatment voluntarily. Neither multiple regression, stepwise regression, nor factor analysis found criminal violence to be predicted by substance abuse, drug dealing activity, or a collection of demographic variables often theoretically linked to violence (i.e., youthfulness, having an early onset of criminal activity, and being male, minority, unmarried, and dually diagnosed). Alternatively, a significant link between poly-drug use and poly-criminality allude to shared underlying causal mechanisms for both substance abuse and violence. *[Article copies available for a fee from The Haworth Document Delivery Service: 1-800-HAWORTH. E-mail address: <docdelivery@haworthpress.com> Website: <http://www.HaworthPress. com> © 2003 by The Haworth Press, Inc. All rights reserved.]*

KEYWORDS Drugs, substance abuse, violence, addict, residential treatment, self-report

A link between drug abuse and criminal violence is often asserted and, in some circles, taken for granted. However, the linkage between substance abuse and violence is complex especially when measured at the individual level. Despite a lack of clear and consistent evidence that drug use produces violent behavior, it is the addict on a "high" and out of control (an image beloved of the entertainment media) that the public has come to fear. The research reported here addresses this fear by examining the empirical relationship between particular substances abused and violent behavior among a seriously addicted population.

PREVIOUS RESEARCH

Drug use has been reported as an antecedent to violence in a few ways. In his tripartite conceptual framework Goldstein (1985) identifies psychopharmacological violence, economic-compulsive violence, and systemic violence all originating from drug involvement. While overlap between each of these perspectives is likely given particular substances, perpetrator motivations, victim characteristics, and social context, Goldstein contends that most drug-generated violence is systemic rather than pharmacologically induced. The research conducted in the present study will be able to demonstrate whether any of the reported violence is due to one or more of the three etiological perspectives outlined by Goldstein. By measuring the frequencies of both self-reported substance abuse and crime commission, a positive association will support the psychopharmacological and the economic-compulsive perspectives, though not enough data exist in this analysis to differentiate between the two. Similarly, a positive association between self-reported drug dealing and self-reported violence may indicate systemic violence.

Considering the biochemical effects of a serious addiction and years of using deceit to hide one's misconduct, the validity of self-reported illegal behavior among addicts is questionable. Reflecting upon his 1977 study of Miami heroin addicts, Inciardi (2001) espouses careful methodological care that was able to uncover far more crime than imagined. However, following the 1977 study he cautioned that poorly designed self-report studies of known substance abusers could produce inaccurate results (Inciardi, 1982). In what Pallone and Hennesey (1996) regard as one of the best designed and executed self-report studies on this matter, McGlothin (1985) concluded that during active addiction, addicts commit more drug-related and property crime but not more violent crime than those who use drugs less frequently. Given the ability of self-reports to reveal far more crime committed than official records, and because privacy rights prohibit access to individuals' official criminal records, data were collected via self-report for the present study.

That most of the literature describing the relationship between drugs and violence actually covers market-generated, or systemic, violence testifies to the lack of confirmatory evidence that consumption of particular drugs causes violent behavior, particularly among addicts who use heavily. In one such study

...ry effort is made to ensure valid data collection. Using feedback from ...s, several revisions had been made to the directions to make the instru-...imple to use and avoid collection of erroneous information. Directions ...so given orally before subjects completed the instrument. All question-...were carefully screened before data entry for contradictory, missing, or ...rdinary answers. If such a case was discovered, clarification was sought ...ly from the subject and if necessary corrections were made.

...r the regression analyses described below, the dependent variable is a ...osite variable, or index, calculated from each case's self-reported scores ...x different measures of violence occurring during the last six months that ...ts spent on the street. These variables are number of aggravated assaults, ...ber of simple assaults, number of robberies, number of domestic assaults, ...ber of stalking incidents/terroristic threats made, and number of illegal ...carrying/possession incidents. Though terroristic threats and gun carrying ...not in and of themselves violent crimes, they are aggressive, potentially vi-...t, and are routine behaviors for those involved in a violent drug market. ...refore, they were included in the dependent variable.

...To be suitable for regression, the dependent variable had to be transformed. ...st, many zero responses skewed the variable to the right. Out of a total sam-...of 184, ninety-five cases were excluded because of no reported violence. ...erefore, regression and factor analyses are based on data from 89 subjects. ...cond, the variable was transformed to its square root to further normalize the ...tribution. Though several transformations were performed, the square root ...nsformation most closely approximated a normal distribution.

...Data were analyzed using SPSS 10.0 with which two stages of regressions ...d a factor analysis were conducted. First, a linear regression of only the vari-...ples that supported each of the three theories was run. Next, a stepwise regres-...on that included all variables appropriate for predicting violence was run. ...he violence index was the dependent variable for both regressions. Finally, a ...actor analysis with varimax rotation was performed to examine the joint cor-...elations of the substance abuse and crime variables.

RESULTS

Out of the total amount of crime committed by these subjects, violence ac-counted for only 13% while drug-related crime accounted for 57% and prop-erty crime, 23% (see Table 1). The remaining 7% were composed of crimes not easily classified in any of these indicies, such as prostitution, gambling, and failure to pay child support. Once these proportions were tabulated it was hypothesized that there would be a significant difference in the self-reported proportions of criminal violence between volunteers and criminal justice ap-pointed clients. Surprisingly, these proportions did not differ at all. For both of these populations, violence was merely 13% of their total self-reported crime.

Farabee, Joshi, and Anglin (2001) analyze data from the Drug Abuse Treat-ment Outcomes Studies (DATOS) and find cocaine, heroin, and the combined use of cocaine and heroin (speedballing) predictive of the frequency of preda-tory crime, yet not predictive when the dependent variable was dichotomized into *any predatory crime/no predatory crime* categories. This may have been due to a relatively weak statistical relationship between drug dependence and predatory crime as measured in their study. Despite the inclusion of ten predic-tors of the frequency of predatory crime, the resultant unadjusted R^2 was merely .23.

Other researchers have similarly found cocaine (Bennett, Tolman, & Rogalski, 1994; Goldstein et al., 1991; Baumer, 1994) and other drugs (Cappel, LeBlanc, & Rosenberg, 1985; Dawkins, 1997) to be predictive of violence, yet evidence to the contrary also exists (Abram & Teplin, 1990; Swartz, 1990). Li, Priu, and MacKenzie (2000) confirmed their hypotheses that drug use is only predictive of property crime while drug dealing is predictive of both property and violent crime.

Given debate over the direct effect of drugs on the commission of violence, another line of research finds that substance abuse and violence share underly-ing causes. In a summary of the current research on the subject, Fishbein (2000) presents a convincing argument that cognitive deficits underlie vio-lence and substance abuse. Dozens of studies highlight dysfunctions in the prefrontal cortexes of violent offenders and substance abusers that negatively affect executive cognitive functioning, giving rise to such problems as impulsivity, poor decision-making ability, disinhibition, inability to assess consequences, and compulsive behavior patterns. Fishbein contends that these are the antecedents to both violence and substance abuse, yet calls for more eti-ological research on these behaviors given the fact that they are both multidetermined and multidimensional.

RESEARCH QUESTIONS

To study the relationship between violence and substance abuse, residents of an inpatient non-hospital drug and alcohol treatment facility were sampled. To maintain a safe environment, it is the facility's policy to not admit clients with official histories of violence. Therefore, insofar as officially recorded vio-lence, the population under study is systematically less violent than a prison population. However, the amount of violence recorded in one's official record is far different than the amount of violence one actually commits. While pre-liminary examinations of the data reveal a surprising amount of violence com-mitted by this addict population, it was accounted for by only about a third of the population. This prompted the general question *why are some of these ad-dicts more violent than others?*

Though this research is largely exploratory and designed to determine if there are any measured variables that would be able to predict the self-reported violence, three plausible hypotheses were evident given theory and previous research. First, and the primary focus of this research, is whether abuse of particular drugs would be predictive of violent behavior. That is, alcohol disinhibits, thus facilitating violence, and drugs such as cocaine, methamphetamine, and PCP have a stimulating effect on the brain, potentially encouraging aggressive behavior (Parker & Rebhun, 1995; Farabee, Joshi, & Anglin, 2001; Li, Priu, & McKenzie, 2000; Cappel, LeBlanc, & Rosenberg, 1985).

A competing hypothesis is that most of the violence would be systemic, or a product of drug-dealing activity (Goldstein, 1985; Li, Priu, & McKenzie, 2000). Besides drug possession, drug dealing is the most common illegal activity reported for this population, and many of the clients are residents of Allentown, Pennsylvania, a medium-sized city with a currently unstable and violent drug market.

Another competing hypothesis is that the violence would be attributable to some combination of demographic variables popularly associated with predatory criminality in subculture and social control theories, the routine activities approach (Cohen & Felson, 1979), and as evidenced in FBI Uniform Crime Statistics. Of particular concern were the effects of youthfulness, having an early onset of criminal activity, and being male, minority, unmarried, and dually diagnosed.

THE SAMPLE

The sample under study consists of 184 current and former residents of Keenan House, a residential drug and alcohol treatment facility in Allentown, Pennsylvania. Keenan House is a modified therapeutic community with a maximum capacity of eighty-five clients. The sample includes only those who have passed through the nearly month-long orientation phase.

Eighty-nine percent (n = 164) of the sample was referred through the criminal justice system while the remaining 11% were referred by either a physician, a family member, another drug and alcohol abuse care provider, or themselves. Sixty-five percent do not have a G.E.D. or high school diploma, and 98% have incomes below poverty level.

Keenan House accepts referrals from local, state, and federal correctional facilities, yet an effort is made to serve residents of Lehigh County and the City of Allentown regardless of where they were previously incarcerated. Largely because two interstate highways bisect the city and because Allentown forms a triangle with nearby Philadelphia and New York City, a steady supply of drugs feeds a sizable substance-abusing population. Though Allentown is the third largest city in Pennsylvania, clients usually know each other, either from the street, jail, or other treatment facilities.

Pennsylvania Client Placement Criteria (PCPC) House clients' drug problems of such severity as to ment. Most are referred to long-term treatment, whic tion. As active addicts, drug use is especially preval During their most recent six months out on the street, tl at least one drug on a daily basis, nearly two different more often basis, and nearly five different drugs over tl

METHODS

After clients complete orientation, they are tested to d ready to become part of the therapeutic community and gra It is at this time that clients complete a questionnaire on pre and criminal behavior. The questionnaire includes, but is following information: frequency of pre-treatment use of th by various routes of administration, primary and secondary times hospitalized due to drug use, frequency of committing ent crimes (drug-related, property, and violent), number of for various crimes, the number of technical violations comm illegal income generated, and years committing crimes asso involvement. Demographic information was collected from c

In accordance with substance abuse program licensure, cli that none of the information can be used against them and will confidential. Following agency confidentiality policy, names lection instrument are limited to first name and last initial. Last nowhere on the self-reported crime and drug use documents and made aware of this.

To help avoid recall problems, responses to self-reported cri use are ordinal, but eight response options for drugs and nine resp for crime allow the data to be treated as interval. Response options variables are 0 = never, 1 = only once, 2 = a few times, 3 = about or 4 = about once every two weeks, 5 = about once a week, 6 = sev week, 7 = every day, and 8 = more than once every day. Response crime commission variables are 0 = never, 1 = once, 2 = two to five six to ten times, 4 = eleven to twenty times, 5 = twenty-one to thirty thirty-one to fifty times, 7 = fifty-one to ninety-nine times, 8 = one h five hundred times, and 9 = more than five hundred times. All inform tains to the clients' most recent six months on the street. The last si chronologically is a less meaningful measure of recent drug use and activity, because many came to treatment directly from incarceration fore, clients are asked to make this information pertain to the last six out on the street prior to their most recent incarceration.

	Volunteer	CJ appointed	Total
□ **Table 1: Criminal Activity of the Sample**			
Drug-related crime	52%	57%	57%
Property crime	26%	23%	23%
Violent crime	13%	13%	13%
Other crime	9%	7%	7%
Number of violent crimes per client annually (total violence index)	31	44	45
Number of violent crimes per client annually (minus gun carrying)	16	19	19

A yearly rate of criminal violence per client calculated from the violence index illustrates that those who are criminal justice-appointed do indeed commit more violent acts annually than volunteers, but not as much as originally expected. By summing the low-end response options for each variable in the violent crime index, the data reveal that volunteers annually commit at minimum 31 violent crimes each, while criminal justice-appointed clients commit at least 44 each. These figures are rather high due to the inclusion of firearm offenses and illegal possessions. Carrying a gun is a daily habit and part of the trade among drug dealers. Thus, by eliminating this variable the figures drop to 16 for volunteers and 19 for criminal justice clients.

Between 16 and 19 stalkings and terroristic threats, robberies, and simple, aggravated, or domestic assaults per client yearly is rather unsettling; especially when one considers that violence is only 13% of the subjects' total self-reported crime. Still surprised in his "(Almost) Twenty-Year Retrospective" of the 1979 findings on heroin and street crime, Inciardi heralds what has been found here: self-report methodology can reveal a much higher rate of crime commission than police incident reports and victimization studies. And while it may be more comforting to know that the bulk of these crimes are daily, habitual low-level drug-related offenses, these data make clear the chronicity of illicit behavior among serious addicts.

Theory-Driven Model Results

Ordinary least squares regression of the violence index failed to support any of the three hypotheses when all predictor variables supportive of each hypotheses were included in the model producing an adjusted R^2 of merely .178 (see Tables 2a & 2b). Being young, male, unmarried, and dually diagnosed were not predictive of violence among this sample. Nor were early onset of criminal activity associated with drug involvement, drug dealing, abusing alcohol, or abus-

☐ *Table 2a: O.L.S. Multiple Regression Model Summary*

R	R Square	Adjusted R Square	Std. Error of the Estimate	Durbin-Watson
.535	.287	.178	1.0716	2.172

☐ *Table 2b: O.L.S. Multiple Regression Model Coefficients*

	Unstandardized Coefficients		Standardized Coefficients		
	B	Std. Error	Beta	t	Sig.
(Constant)	3.280	.659		4.974	.000
Sex: 0 = male, 1 = female	−.110	.356	−.035	−.309	.758
Race/ethnicity: 0 = nonwhite, 1 = white	−.322	.277	−.133	−1.161	.249
Dual diagnosis: 0 = no, 1 = yes	2.4E-02	.292	.009	.083	.934
Marital status: 0 = not married, 1 = married	8.7E-02	.573	.016	.151	.880
Age	−1.7E-02	.018	−.122	−.934	.354
Age of onset of crime associated with drug involvement	−3.1E-02	.019	−.197	−1.607	.112
Drug dealing	3.8E-02	.039	.116	.993	.324
Cocaine or crack use	−1.7E-02	.026	−.075	−.651	.517
Drinking casually or to intoxication	3.1E-02	.030	.113	1.061	.292
Methamphetamine use**	.170	.052	.406	3.256	.002
PCP use	3.0E-02	.069	.053	.441	.661

Dependent variable: Square root of violence index; non-zero values included only.
** = $p \leq .01$.

ing most of the stimulants generally charged with exciting violent behavior. In this analysis, methamphetamine abuse was the sole statistically significant predictor of violence, yet accounted for far too little variance to be noteworthy.

Stepwise Regression Results

The stepwise procedure (see Tables 3a & 3b) produced three models, the most predictive of which yielded an adjusted R^2 of only .306 and was composed of only three predictor variables: poly-criminality (the variety of crimes

□ **Table 3a: Stepwise Regression Model Summary**

R	R Square	Adjusted R Square	Std. Error of the Estimate
.574	.330	.306	1.0077

□ **Table 3b: Stepwise Regression Model Coefficients**

	Unstandardized Coefficients		Standardized Coefficients		
	B	Std. Error	Beta	t	Sig.
(Constant)	1.392	.328		4.238	.000
Variety of crimes reported (minus violence variables)***	.177	.040	.407	4.369	.000
Crack/freebase use*	−8.E-02	.034	−.205	−2.264	.026
Use of methamphetamine, not injected**	.212	.071	.281	2.964	.004

Dependent variable: Square root of violence index; non-zero values included only.
*** = $p \leq .001$; ** = $p \leq .01$; * = $p \leq .05$.

reported minus violent variables), crack/freebase use, and non-injection use of methamphetamine. These findings indicate that the form of a drug ingested and its route of administration may be important factors in predicting violence. The specific use of crack/freebase, rather than any form and route of administration of cocaine as tested in the theory driven model (see Tables 2a & 2b), is, albeit slightly, of more predictive value. The same holds true for methamphetamine use. Although both stimulants, crack and methamphetamine, were statistically significant predictors as hypothesized from previous research, they were of minimal predictive value.

Factor Analysis Results

Two measures of the data's suitability for factor analysis show the procedure to be acceptable for the data. The Kaiser, Meyer, Olkin (KMO) Measure of Sampling Adequacy finds 79.4% of the variance among these individual variables is common variance, indicating the presence of underlying factors. The Bartlett Test of Sphericity is significant at the .000 level indicating the presence of significant relationships among the variables. These statistics offer sufficient confidence for interpreting the following factor analytical results.

Nine factors were produced from thirty-three self-reported drug use and crime variables that accounted for roughly 67% of the total variance. Due to too few non-zero responses, arson, and use of inhalants, amphetamines, street methadone, steroids, and designer drugs other than MDMA were excluded from the analysis. Partial correlation values less than .365 were suppressed from the rotated component matrix for the reader to more easily distinguish independent factors. Although a small number of variables that successfully loaded on one factor were partially correlated with another factor at greater than .365, these values were deleted from Table 4 to further help distinguish factors from one another.

Two significant findings are immediately evident in Table 4. First, none of the six violence variables loaded onto factors containing any drug use variables. This demonstrates the absence of a statistical relationship between substance abuse and violence overall, and the absence of statistical relationships between specific forms of violence and specific drugs abused. Second, all six violence variables partitioned off into just two distinct factors. Factor one contains aggravated assault, simple assault, firearms offenses, and robbery creating a factor nearly exclusive to aggressive, violent activity. The variables measuring stalking/menacing/terroristic threats and domestic assault appropriately loaded together on factor six. These two variables are likely bedmates and are clearly distinct from the other violence variables as they characterize a domineering, abusive partner, rather than one whose violence may be instrumental to other criminal activity.

Readers should be careful to interpret factor analysis findings with caution. If substance abuse and violence share an underlying cause and if factor analysis is supposed to unearth underlying factors, one may expect to see significant mingling of the violence and drug use variables within the factors. Such an assumption would be inaccurate for two reasons. First, underlying cause and underlying factors are not equivalent. Factors merely illustrate the joint correlations among variables and do not imply underlying causality. Second, whether substance abuse and violence share the same causal mechanism does not imply that it will manifest both problems or either problem in the same way.

CONCLUSIONS

These findings reveal a weak relationship between substance abuse and violence among this addict population and, clearly, not all addicts are violent. In fact, most of this population is not. Many cases had to be excluded from the analyses because of no reported recent violence. It appears that the violence committed by an addict population may stem more from lifestyle characteristics (characteristics unfortunately not measured in this analysis) or some other general propensity toward deviance rather than from particular demographic variables, drug dealing, or drug use itself. Such lifestyle or deviance characteristics may also underlie both violent behavior and drug use among this population.

☐ **Table 4: Factor Analysis of Substance Abuse and Crime Variables**

	Component								
	1	2	3	4	5	6	7	8	9
Aggravated assaults & batteries	.763								
Simple assaults & batteries	.687								
Manufacturing illegal drugs	.662								
Firearm offenses/illegal possessions	.620								
Robberies	.553								
Illegal gambling offenses	.435								
Burglaries		.806							
Vandalism offenses		.741							
Auto thefts		.612							
Fencing offenses		.599							
Other thefts (e.g., larceny)		.574							
Forgery or fraud offenses		.450							
Prostitution-related offenses		.365							
Minor tranquilizer use			.830						
Codeine, Percoset, Morphine, Demerol use			.771						
Xanax or other benzodiazepine use			.708						
Methamphetamine use			.488						
Possession of illegal drugs				.834					
Purchasing illegal drugs				.806					
Dealing drugs				.686					
Marijuana/hashish use				.569					
MDMA (ecstasy) use					.794				
DUI/DWI offenses					.526				
PCP use					.433				

| | Table 4 (continued) | | | | | | | | |
| | Component | | | | | | | | |
	1	2	3	4	5	6	7	8	9
Stalking, menacing, or making terroristic threats						.723			
Domestic assaults & batteries						.670			
Embezzlement offenses						.498			
Snorting or smoking heroin							.824		
Using heroin & cocaine together							.683		
Drinking casually or to intoxication								.574	
Injecting heroin								−.541	
Cocaine or crack use									.712
Failure to pay child support									.646

Extraction method: Principal Component Analysis
Rotation method: Varimax with Kaiser Normalization

Interestingly, the strongest predictor of violence was poly-criminality, the variety of different crimes for which commission is reported. While the regression analysis excluded the redundant violent variables to eliminate overlap between the predictor and dependent variables, a significant correlation was found between the full poly-criminality variable (violent variables included) and poly-drug use (Pearson's $r = .526$, $n = 188$). This finding is particularly true among female clients ($r = .642$, $n = 40$).

A solid correlation between poly-drug use and poly-criminality, yet very little evidence of a causal connection between substance abuse and crime is indicative of general deviance, and that these phenomena share an underlying cause. The common antecedent could be a pervasive deviant lifestyle and routine activities, opportunism, cognitive impairment, or some combination of these.

That violence is poorly predicted by drug use calls into question the rationality of the public's fear of addicts and the efficacy of drug-related mandatory minimum sentences. While a small subset of addicts is indeed violent and is probably safest while incarcerated, these data indicate that their violence is not a product of their substance abusing and dealing habits. Rather, their substance abuse is one more expression of their general propensity toward antisocial behavior. It is likely that public safety would be better served by targeting those who engage in violence, property offenses, drug offenses, and substance abuse combined, rather than the act of substance abuse alone.

REFERENCES

Abram, K. M. & Teplin, L. A. (1990). Drug disorder, mental illness, and violence. In M. De La Rosa, E. Y. Lambert, & B. Gropper (Eds.), *Drugs and Violence: Causes, Correlates, and Consequences* (pp. 222-238). Rockville, MD: National Institute of Drug Abuse.

Baumer, E. (1994). Poverty, crack, and crime: A cross-city analysis. *Journal of Research in Crime and Delinquency*, 31(3), 311-327.

Bennett, L. W., Tolman, R. M., & Rogalski, C. J. (1994). Domestic abuse by male alcohol and drug addicts. *Violence and Victims*, 9(4), 359-368.

Cappel, H., LeBlanc, A. E., & Rosenberg, M. (1985). Alcohol, drugs, and assaultive crime: Pharmacological considerations. In M. H. Ben-Aron, S. J. Hucker, & C. D. Webster (Eds.), *Clinical Criminology: The Assessment and Treatment of Criminal Behaviour* (pp. 131-156). Toronto, CAN.

Cohen, L. E., & Felson, M. (1979). Social changes and crime rate trends: A routine activity approach. *American Sociological Review*, 44, 588-608.

Dawkins, M. P. (1997). Drug use and violent crime among adolescents. *Adolescence*, 32(126), 395-405.

Farabee, D., Joshi V., & Anglin, M. D. (2001). Addiction careers and criminal specialization. *Crime and Delinquency*, 47(2), 196-220.

Fishbein, D. (2000). Neuropsychological function, drug abuse, and violence. *Criminal Justice and Behavior*, 27(2), 139-159.

Goldstein, Paul J. (1985). The drugs/violence nexus: A tripartite conceptual framework. *Journal of Drug Issues*, 15(4), 493-506.

Inciardi, J. A. & Pottieger A. E. (2001). Drug use and street crime in Miami: An (Almost) twenty-year retrospective. In J. A. Inciardi & K. McElrath (Eds.), *The American Drug Scene: An Anthology Third Edition* (pp. 319-341). Los Angeles, CA: Roxbury Publishing Company.

McGolothin, W. H. (1985). Distinguishing effects from concomitants of drug use: The case of crime. In Lee N. Robins (Ed.), *Studying Drug Abuse: Series in Psychosocial Epidemiology, VI* (pp. 153-172). New Brunswick, NJ: Rutgers University Press.

Swartz, James A. (1990) *Cocaine and opiates: Prevalence estimates of their use by arrestees and a theoretical and empirical investigation of their relationship to the commission of violent crime.* Ann Arbor, MI: University Microfilms International.

AUTHOR'S NOTE

At the time of preparation of this report, Eric Workowski was a researcher at Treatment Trends, Inc. in Allentown, PA. Presently, he is an osteoporosis specialty representative with Merck & Co., Inc. His research interests include substance abuse treatment effectiveness and the relationship between drugs and crime.

Address correspondence to Eric Workowski, Merck & Co., Inc., 100 Knittle Rd., Kutztown, PA 19530.

Treating Substance Abusers in Correctional Contexts: New Understandings, New Modalities. Pp. 123-137.
10.1300/J076v37n03_07

RSAT Programs
for Young Offenders in California:
A Descriptive Study

ANGELA HEGAMIN

California State University, Los Angeles

DAVID FARABEE

University of California, Los Angeles

ABSTRACT The present study sought to identify drug treatment issues unique to corrections-based residential drug treatment programs for youthful offenders. Based upon qualitative data collected from program administrators and wards at three institution-based substance abuse treatment programs in California, four themes were identified which hold important implications for the delivery of substance abuse treatment services in these settings: screening/assessment, quality and intensity of services, appropriateness of program elements, and anticipated problems once paroled. Our data revealed a substantial amount of overlap in perceptions shared by program administrators and wards, as well as across programs. Of particular concern were low treatment intensity within the institution and insufficient social support upon release. *[Article copies available for a fee from The Haworth Document Delivery Service: 1-800-HAWORTH. E-mail address: <docdelivery@ haworthpress.com> Website: <http://www.HaworthPress.com> © 2003 by The Haworth Press, Inc. All rights reserved.]*

KEYWORDS Incarcerated youths, youthful offenders, adolescents, corrections-based treatment, drug abuse

In 1994, Congress passed the Violent Crime Control and Law Enforcement Act, creating the Residential Substance Abuse Treatment for State Prisoners (RSAT) Formula Grant Program. This program provides grants to states to assist in the development or enhancement of drug treatment programs for youthful offenders. While it is clear that the RSAT funding has resulted in the rapid expansion of these programs throughout the United States, the extent to which this initiative will lead to a reduction in substance abuse among youthful parolees has yet to be determined. Moreover, process data documenting the implementation of RSAT programs for youthful offenders are absent from the literature.

The provision of substance abuse treatment to youthful offenders in these programs entails a number of challenges, unique to both the correctional setting and the drug treatment milieu. Aside from managing the day-to-day delivery of drug treatment services, prison-based programs must comply with the custodial regulations of the host institution. In addition to performing these institutional functions, correctional staff employed by drug treatment programs must ensure that their caseloads receive therapeutic interventions on drug abuse (e.g., individual or group counseling sessions). Moreover, whether custody and treatment duties are performed by the same or separate staff there is a common perception that security and treatment goals are conflictive (Leukefeld, Gallego, & Farabee, 1997), with the former, by necessity, taking priority (Morrissey, Steadman, & Kilburn, 1983).

The present study sought to identify drug treatment issues unique to corrections-based residential drug treatment programs for youthful offenders. In California, RSAT funds were used to augment existing drug treatment services to include additional psychological screening and assessment resources, drug testing equipment and supplies, staff training, additional counseling hours, and release time to improve quality and quantity of counseling services, and enhanced linkages between of institutional and field parole components. The resultant residential treatment programs consisted of group counseling sessions led by correctional counselors, individual counseling on an "as needed" basis provided by a psychologist, and, for wards who were minors, drug education classes based on the Hazelden Design for Living Curriculum administered by education staff. Wards were referred to drug treatment by the parole board at the recommendation of psychological staff at regional reception centers. A total of 855 RSAT beds were available at the time of the study.

A process evaluation was undertaken beginning in 1998 to determine the extent to which program activities and services had achieved the RSAT enhancements and to assess the effectiveness of each program with regard to its implementation. As part of this evaluation, semi-structured interviews were conducted with administrative staff, and focus groups were conducted with wards at three California RSAT Programs. The findings of this study derive from these interviews and focus groups. Because the samples, procedures, and analyses for the program administrator interviews and ward focus groups differed, the methods and results are described separately below.

STUDY 1:
SEMI-STRUCTURED PROGRAM
ADMINISTRATOR INTERVIEWS

Materials and Methods

Sample. Semi-structured interviews were conducted with a purposive sample of drug treatment program administrators at three correctional youth institutions in California. These programs represented both the northern and southern regions of the state. Since this study sought to measure perceptions of program administrators providing oversight to the each of these programs, those recruited were selected based upon the extent to which their positions entailed administrative tasks designed to ensure implementation of program activities. Of the 19 individuals approached for recruitment into the study, all agreed to participate. The resultant sample was comprised of program directors (n = 3), treatment staff supervisors (n = 6), psychologists (n = 3), institutional parole agents (n = 4), senior counseling staff (n = 2) and a school principal at these three youth correctional facilities. Most had worked for the drug treatment program for at least one year, and those who were new to the program were not new to the institution.

Procedures. Items comprising the semi-structured interview schedule covered a range of program implementation issues, including successes of the drug treatment program, barriers to implementation and recommendations for improvement. Interviews were conducted by members of the research team, including 3 senior researchers, 1 research associate and 2 research assistants. Interviews were conducted on-site at each facility and took approximately 1 hour to complete. At the beginning of each interview, participants were informed that their individual-level responses would remain confidential but that, for research purposes, their aggregate responses to interview items would be reported. Every participant gave his or her permission. Table 1 lists the questions posed to program administrators.

Analysis. Responses to interview questions were recorded verbatim by a member of the research team. At the conclusion of each interview, these notes were reviewed for accuracy and revised as necessary by the interviewer. Interview notes were subsequently typed, and the resultant transcripts were prepared for manual coding.

Transcript data were analyzed in a three-stage process. First, each transcript was manually coded by two senior researchers and cross-coded according to the broad themes established *a priori* by the semi-structured interview schedule. These codes were then reviewed to determine the degree to which both raters agreed on the initial classification of item responses. The transcripts were

□ ***Table 1: Semi-Structured Interview Schedule Items***

How long have you worked for the drug treatment program?

Do you enjoy your job?

Have you ever done work like this before? If so, where? For how long?

What are your educational credentials?

What "enhancements" (e.g., additional personnel or other resources, supplies and materials, etc.) has your program been able to add as a result of the RSAT grant? [Please list.]

What have been some of the successes so far in the RSAT enhanced program?

What have been some of the barriers to implementing the RSAT enhanced program so far?

What are the main objectives of this project? What are the secondary objectives?

How will the program lead to the achievement of these objectives?

How is the communication between treatment staff and CYA administration? (i.e., Do you receive information from CYA administration in a timely manner?) [Examples, if any.]

In your opinion, what have been some of the start-up plans or activities that have been successful?

In your opinion, what have been some of the start-up plans or activities that have *not* been successful?

If you had to plan a program like this, what would you do differently?

What have been some of the problems that have come up and have been handled well?

What have been some of the problems that have come up that were *not* handled well?

Overall, how would you describe the working conditions at this program?

What formal substance abuse training have you received?

Have you received enough training? If not what areas need attention?

What training has been most beneficial?

Is the physical environment appropriate for this program? Why or why not?

How will you know the program is successful? Do you have your own measure of success? If so, what does your measure include?

Do you see any short-term outcomes at the program level and at the client level which indicate that programs are on track? [Please give examples.]

then formatted for electronic coding in QSR NUD*IST 4. Second, using the broad themes identified in the manual coding stage, text from the transcripts was organized into coding categories or "nodes" (Maietta & Gnida, 1999) to prepare the data for multiple analysis of identical bodies of text. Using QSR NUD*IST 4, each transcript was then recoded internally by two research assistants, each of whom reviewed all transcripts independently. The inter-rater reliability attained in this process was 74%. In the third and final stage of analysis, text-based searches were undertaken to identify themes common to all 19 interviews. The resultant themes were classified into the four categories discussed below. Where appropriate, verbatim responses to particular interview questions are noted to illustrate the contextual dimensions of the item.

Results

Screening for program eligibility. Most program administrators believed that the process by which eligibility for program enrollment was determined was sufficiently sensitive to detect individuals in need of substance abuse treatment. However, some respondents noted the substantial influence of the Youthful Offender Parole Board (YOPB) in the decision to refer wards to drug treatment.

> About 85% of wards are appropriate. The remaining 15% come from YOPB recommendations that are inappropriate.

> They are here because they have to be here. They are Board-ordered. You'll get a lot of surface conformity. A lot of wards come here because they don't want to "max out." They can get out sooner if they come here.

The involvement of the Board in the screening process had, in some instances, resulted in the placement of wards not suitable for the program (e.g., dually diagnosed wards or wards not motivated to participate in treatment), contributing to the depletion of limited program resources to provide services to wards with broad and complex range of needs. Moreover, these individuals were often disruptive to the treatment process in which appropriately placed wards willingly participated.

> Lots of dual diagnosis. This is fine, but the YCCs [youth correctional counselors] need more training for this population.

> We have hard core drugs users, psychopaths, antisocial personality disorders. We get some "strange wards," sometimes psychotic every once in a while.

Psychological assessment. Many respondents expressed satisfaction with existing psychological assessment protocols used by their programs. But several were either unaware of these protocols or had supervised staff who simply did not use psychological data to customize treatment to the ward's individual needs. A single, standardized assessment procedure had not been adopted across these programs.

They [the assessments] are sufficient. They are done at entry into our program. Wards are regularly assessed as part of their program.

I would like to see this information sooner and in a more understandable format. We need something shorter. We need one person to do just assessments. I can't assess everybody.

I am unaware of any treatment assessments.

The psychologist sees them. Her assessments are not yet linked with treatment, and only rarely is she involved in wards' case conferences.

Staff training. Many administrators indicated a personal need for additional training to enhance their ability to perform their jobs. In addition, respondents expressed a need for training for youth correctional counselors in their programs, particularly those newly hired or assigned to the programs. The desire for training for counseling staff was reported by several respondents and is evidenced by the following verbatim responses.

Counselors are coming in with no skills from non-treatment programs.

Prior training or experience is not a requirement for the job. Need to train the YCCs more in doing groups.

They have a lack of knowledge of basic counseling skills.

Newly hired counselors come from the Academy and aren't well versed on counseling skills. They need more training on counseling techniques and on how to counsel. They should also have ongoing training on drug counseling, continuously.

We've brought in a lot of new staff over the past year, and we've just thrown them to the lions. We've given them materials and left them to do what they can. They need more training on how to do small groups; existing resources are limited.

Counseling services. Most respondents believed that wards had not received a sufficient amount of individual counseling while in the program. Reasons cited for this deficiency included lack of staff training, excessive workloads, institutional policies that prevent wards from being excused from school to participate in counseling sessions and inappropriate use of time allotted for counseling. Conversely, a majority of those interviewed believed that wards in their programs had received a sufficient amount of group counseling, although one respondent felt that the quality of the groups could be enhanced by providing the counseling staff more training and by making groups smaller.

> YCCs are too busy. Wards want it but can't get it. I wish I could be compensated for coming in early and staying late. I would use this time to work with wards individually.

> Day-to-day operations take so much time and energy that the YCCs simply can't do it [provide individual counseling].

> They could use a lot more [individual counseling]. They get enough groups. In a prison setting, people will not be as open [in groups] as they would be in individual sessions.

> Most counseling is on a group basis. Those with special needs are given individual counseling, and they have to be very special needs to get the counseling.

> Groups happen regularly but are often rushed since they might start late but are required to end on time.

STUDY 2: WARD FOCUS GROUPS

Materials and Methods

Sample. In addition to interviews with administrative staff, focus groups were conducted with wards at each of the three program sites. The purpose of these groups was to solicit wards' opinions regarding the treatment program and the manner in which services were delivered. Table 2 lists the questions posed to focus group participants. Prospective participants were identified from current population rosters at each facility. The criteria for stratification included ward sex and living unit; the former criterion was necessary due to institutional policies prohibiting the integration of male and female wards, and the latter was undertaken strategically to ensure that particular living units were neither over- nor underrepresented. A total of four focus groups (3 with males, 1 with females) were conducted.

In keeping with the requirements set forth by the UCLA Human Subject Protection Committee (HSPC), only wards 18 years of age and older were eligible for participation in focus groups. However, it is unlikely that the exclusion of minors from the focus groups posed a significant threat to the generalizeability of findings, given that minors constituted only 3.5% of the wards at the 3 programs studied. Table 3 depicts the characteristics of respondents participating in focus groups.

☐ *Table 2: Focus Group Questionnaire Items*

1. What part of the drug treatment program do you find most useful?

2. How would you describe your relationship with the treatment team supervisors? Counselors? Parole agents?

3. How often do you meet with the same counselor on a regular basis?

4. Have you had the same counselor throughout your entire stay in the program? If not, please explain.

5. Can you relate to the experiences of the people shown in the videos or other materials (e.g., workbooks and other handouts) used in the program?

6. How could the videos and or written materials be improved?

7. What problems have you had during your stay in the program? Have they been adequately addressed? If not, why not?

8. What successes or achievements have you had as result of being in the program?

9. What problems do you foresee in dealing with drugs once you are on parole? How could parole agents or others in your community help you deal with these problems?

10. Do you have suggestions for improving or changing the program?

☐ *Table 3: Characteristics of Focus Group Participants (N = 32)*

Mean Age (SD)	19.8 (1.7)
Female (%)	25
Primary Drug of Abuse	
Marijuana	15
Alcohol	3
Methamphetamine	11
Hallucinogens	1
Heroin	2
Mean Number of Times in Treatment (SD)	1.7 (0.8)
Mean Number of Months in Program (SD)	10.9 (10.4)

Procedures. Focus groups were conducted by a facilitator and a notetaker, each of whom had received formal training in this form of data collection. To ensure that wards did not feel coerced into participating in the focus group, initial groups of 16-20 wards at each site were convened so that focus group facilitators could describe the purpose of the study and invite the wards to participate. Wards were given an information sheet describing the purpose of the study and indicating that participation in the focus group was strictly voluntary. Wards were then asked to express their interest in participating by checking "yes" or "no" on the second page of the form and returning that page to the research staff member. Forms were collected by members of the research team, who subsequently removed the sheets of those not wishing to participate and randomly selected 8 sheets from among the remaining wards expressing an interest in participating. Response rates ranged from 75% to 100%, depending upon the program site. Thus, for each group, 8 participants were chosen and agreed to participate.

Focus groups were conducted on-site at each facility and took approximately 1.5 hours to complete. At the beginning of each group, participants were informed that their responses would not be associated with individual identifiers and that all information disclosed during the group would remain confidential, with the exception of data reported in aggregate form for the purpose of research and information that the research team was legally mandated to report (e.g., reports of child abuse). All participants agreed to participate under these terms. At the conclusion of the groups at two program sites, candy bars were provided to participants as reimbursements for their participation in the group; the remaining site did not permit distribution of candy bars to wards in their program.

Analysis. Responses to focus group questions were recorded verbatim by the notetaker. At the conclusion of each group, these notes were reviewed for accuracy and reconciled with general notes recorded by the facilitator. The resultant notes were subsequently typed and prepared for manual coding.

Similar to semi-structured interview data, focus group data were analyzed in a three-stage process. First, each transcript was manually coded by a senior researcher and cross-coded according to the broad themes established *a priori* by the focus group protocol. The transcripts were then formatted for electronic coding in QSR NUD*IST 4. Second, using the broad themes identified in the manual coding stage, text from the transcripts was organized into coding categories or "nodes" (Maietta & Gnida, 1999) to prepare the data for multiple analysis of identical bodies of text. Using QSR NUD*IST 4, each transcript was then recoded internally by a senior researcher and a research assistant, each of whom reviewed all transcripts independently. The inter-rater reliability attained during this process was 78%. In the third and final stage of analysis, text-based searches were undertaken to identify themes common to all 4 focus groups. The resultant themes were classified into the three categories discussed below. As in the case of administrator interviews, verbatim responses to focus group questions are noted to provide context.

Results

Desired components. Many participants expressed a desire for peer-led in-terventions (e.g., Alcoholics Anonymous [AA] or Narcotics Anonymous [NA]) and testimonials from other persons in recovery. One ward resented the incorporation of religious principles into the treatment curriculum. Other par-ticipants felt that the programs' transitional component was essential to their success once paroled.

> I think using groups like AA and NA who can give you testimonial should be a regular part of meetings. I resent getting a college student fresh out and having them tell me what I can or can't do as far as using drugs. They have no idea what my tolerance level is. Now don't get me wrong. I have no problem with college people. Both my parents are grad-uates. But I need people with life experience to tell me like it is.

> I think they [the program] should have wards who were once here and who have made it on the outside and beat their addictions come back and talk to us. I would respect that more coming from them.

> I would like to see individual participants giving lectures and surveys. I think letting a ward take control of a group meeting and open the forum for discussion would be a good thing. Maybe some type of system in place for drug testing can be used a reward. They come up clean so many times, they can lead a group. I ask myself how can we be expected to learn if we are not part of the solution.

> I think pre-parole . . . helps you to learn about going on job interviews and filling out applications. Tells you how to dress. Makes me feel like I have a chance of going someplace and not looking stupid trying to fill out an application like I'm screwed up.

Program materials. A majority of participants felt that the videos used in the programs were outdated or unrealistic. Others indicated that it was difficult to relate to the terminology used in the videos or to the religious principles pro-moted in the curriculum. Some believed that videos could be easily replaced with inexpensive videotape recordings of television programs focused on sub-stance abuse or low-cost documentaries developed by current wards. Books and handouts were felt to be outdated and in poor condition.

> I don't like the way they [the videos] use actors. They have not been in our shoes. They have no street smarts. They are like reading from a script. They don't know where you are coming from. They are like giv-ing you advice they read out of some book and expect you to take it.

I can't relate to the vocabulary, and I don't like the fact that most of the stuff that is being taught is religion based. I feel like they are trying to force religion into this.

The teacher sometimes uses real movies that we can relate to. We dread going through the book, but the teacher now has us go through it in alternative ways.

Problems once paroled. Several participants were concerned about their ability to remain drug-free once paroled. Some felt that their most difficult challenge would result from returning to communities in which drug use is widespread. Others feared that drug use by family members or friends would hasten their relapse to drug use. However, a few participants believed that, ultimately, their decision to remain abstinent would rest upon their personal ability to resist drug use.

The only problem I see is getting out and kicking it with the homies. I live where I live, and that is not going to change, so I'm going right back to where I came out of. I think getting a job will probably be the hardest thing for me.

I think there should be some type of follow up to the drug program when you get out to make you stay clean. I know I am going to have to piss in a cup for tests for my parole agent, but if I am getting no other type of counseling, then it is going to be harder to want to stay clean.

I am worried about going back to where I live at and wanting to fit in and then I am going to use again and then I'm headed straight back here.

For me, it is like my family is all on drugs. It's kind of hard to explain. My dad is a flake. He don't care what I do. I just feel like if he don't care, I am just going to do something stupid. My mom and sister are crack addicts. They use that shit all the time. They are always whacked out. I mean all day. They would be giving me drugs.

DISCUSSION

The primary goal of the present study was to identify issues affecting the provision of substance abuse treatment services in youth correctional settings. Although these data were collected from facilities in the same state, we believe the fact that they were collected from multiple program sites and from male and female wards enhances the external validity of the findings. To further extend the external validity of this study, the topics presented in this paper were limited to those identified across the three programs evaluated, rather than findings specific to any single site. After making this distinction, four themes emerged which hold important implications for the delivery of substance abuse treatment in youth correctional settings: screening/assessment, quality and intensity of services, appropriateness of program elements, and anticipated problems once paroled.

Although most program administrators believed that the initial screening and referral process was adequate, some expressed frustration that these determinations were made by the parole board rather than by trained clinicians. In some cases, this approach had led to the inappropriate referral of wards who either did not have serious substance abuse problems or had significant co-occurring mental disorders that affected their amenability to treatment. Indeed, the tendency to rely on limited criteria (e.g., any lifetime use, involvement in drug sales) to determine need for treatment has been identified in other juvenile justice (Hoge, 1999) and adult correctional systems (Farabee et al., 1999). The effects of inadequate screening can be quite serious, with inappropriate referrals consuming limited treatment resources that might otherwise have been applied to those with more severe drug problems (Knight, Simpson, & Hiller, 1999).

Once at the treatment facility, the administration and use of psychological assessments varied considerably by program. While some program administrators were satisfied with the psychological assessments conducted on newly admitted wards, many were either unaware that such assessments were being conducted or were not taking this information into account when developing treatment plans. This lack of emphasis on specific wards' needs in developing treatment plans is unfortunate, given that dynamic characteristics of offenders have been shown to be more predictive of future offending than static characteristics such as gender and race (Gendreau, Goggin, & Paparozzi, 1996; Motiuk, 1998).

The issues raised concerning treatment intensity can be divided into two dimensions: *quality*, which can be most directly linked to training; and *quantity*, which is associated with competing job duties and caseloads. The majority of program administrators voiced a need for additional training, both for themselves and for front line correctional counselors. Moreover, whereas recovering addicts or ex-offenders comprise the majority of treatment staff in community-based programs, hiring policies for youth correctional counselors disallow hiring of staff with prior drug use and/or criminal histories. While this policy may be justified, it results in a treatment staff with minimal formal training in substance abuse and virtually no personal experience from which to draw. As a consequence, a number of wards questioned the credibility of correctional counselors and their ability to understand the problems faced by the wards in their daily lives. With regard to the quantity of treatment provided, most of the program administrators reported that the correctional counselors could only provide counseling after they had completed their custody duties.

Given that their caseloads were virtually identical in size to those of correctional officers on general population facilities, treatment activities were often given short shrift or neglected altogether. This tendency for custody goals to eclipse treatment goals has been identified for adult correctional programs as well (Morrissey, Steadman, & Kilburn, 1983).

When asked to describe what additional components they believed would improve the program, several wards expressed a desire to hear testimonials from recovering addicts and ex-offenders. This could occur through AA/NA meetings or through establishing a mechanism to recruit guest speakers with similar backgrounds to the wards who could share their accounts of their own recovery. Wards appeared to be very sensitive to the differences between themselves and actors in the drug education videos. Many of the wards reported that they found the actors to be "fake" or from such different social backgrounds that their testimonies lacked relevance to their own lives. In short, virtually all of the wards expressed a strong preference for personal testimonies from persons in recovery from drug addiction with similar backgrounds over videos or written materials.

Finally, and perhaps of greatest importance to sustaining gains achieved during the institutional phase of treatment, wards shared a number of concerns about their ability to abstain from using drugs once released from custody. Drug use is commonplace among wards' peers and, in many cases, immediate families. Although parolees from these treatment programs are required to submit to regular drug testing and to participate in some form of post-release drug counseling, all of the wards were keenly aware of the powerful temptations they would face back in their own communities. Indeed, there is evidence that pre- and during-treatment characteristics of adolescent substance abuse treatment clients fail to account for a substantial amount of variance in post-treatment outcomes, suggesting that factors in the adolescents' post-release environment play a critical role in treatment outcomes (Braukmann et al., 1985). Furthermore, the treatment evaluation literature concerning adult substance-abusing offenders suggests that community-based treatment after release from prison may be more essential to recovery than treatment received while in prison (Inciardi et al., 1997; Knight et al., 1997; Prendergast, Wellisch, & Wong, 1996; Wexler, Falkin, Lipton, & Rosenblum, 1992).

The qualitative data summarized in the present paper identify several critical issues for treating adolescents with substance abuse problems in correctional settings: screening/assessment, quality and intensity of services, appropriateness of program elements, and anticipated problems once paroled. The issues that were identified were consistent across programs and, in many cases, between program administrators and wards. Furthermore, as we have demonstrated in the present section, variations of these same themes have been reported elsewhere in the research literature. The findings from this exploratory study emerged through qualitative interviews and focus groups with both providers and recipients of drug treatment services. We believe that the themes identified in the present study could have relevance for future studies of youthful offender treatment. Moreover, for policy makers, clinicians, and researchers desiring to penetrate the "black box" of the treatment process, qualitative explorations of this nature can be an invaluable tool.

REFERENCES

Braukmann, C.J., Bedlington, M.M., Belden, B.D., Braukmann, B.P.D., Husted, J.J., Ramp, K.K., & Wolf, M.M. (1985). Effects of a community-based group home treatment program on male juvenile offenders' use and abuse of drugs and alcohol. *American Journal of Drug and Alcohol Abuse, 11*, 249-278.

Farabee, D., Prendergast, M.L., Cartier, J., Wexler, W., Knight, K., & Anglin, M.D. (1999). Barriers to implementing effective correctional drug treatment programs. *The Prison Journal, 79*, 150-162.

Gendreau, P., Goggin, C., & Paparozzi, M. (1996). Principles of effective assessment for community corrections. *Federal Probation, 60*, 64-70.

Hoge, R.D. (1999). An expanded role for psychological assessments in juvenile justice systems. *Criminal Justice and Behavior, 26*, 251-266.

Inciardi, J.A., Martin, S.S., Butzin, C.F., Hooper, R.M., & Harrison, L.D. (1997). An effective model of prison-based treatment for drug-involved offenders. *Journal of Drug Issues, 27*(2), 261-278.

Knight, K., Simpson, D.D., & Hiller, M. (1999/2000). Three-year reincarceration outcomes for in-prison therapeutic community treatment in Texas. *Prison Journal, 79*, 337-351.

Knight, K., Simpson, D.D., Chatham, L.R., & Camacho, L.M. (1997). An assessment of prison-based drug treatment: Texas' in-prison therapeutic community program. *Journal of Offender Rehabilitation, 24*(3/4), 75-100.

Leukefeld, C.G., Gallego, M.A., & Farabee, D. (1997). Drugs, crime, and HIV. *Substance Use & Misuse, 32*, 749-756.

Maietta, R.C. & Gnida, J.J. (1999). *QSR NUD*IST 4 Workshop Materials Pack.* Patchogue, New York: Research Talk Consultation and Training.

Morrissey, J.P., Steadman, H.J., & Kilburn, H.C. (1983). Organizational issues in the delivery of jail mental health services. *Research in Community and Mental Health, 3*, 291-317.

Prendergast, M.L., Wellisch, J., & Wong, M.M. (1996). Residential treatment for women parolees following prison-based drug treatment: Treatment experiences, needs and services, outcomes. *Prison Journal, 76*(3), 253-274.

Violent Crime Control and Law Enforcement Act, 42 U.S.C. § 3796ff (1994).

Wexler, H.K., Falkin, G.P., Lipton, D.S., & Rosenblum, A.B. (1992). Outcome evaluation of a prison therapeutic community for substance abuse treatment. In C.G Leukefeld & F.M. Tims (Eds.), *Drug Abuse Treatment in Prisons and Jails.* NIDA Research Monograph 118, pp. 156-175. Rockville, MD: National Institute on Drug Abuse.

AUTHORS' NOTES

At the time of this study, Angela Hegamin was an assistant research social ecologist at the UCLA Drug Abuse Research Center in Los Angeles, California. She is now an assistant professor of Health Science at California State University, Los Angeles. Her primary research interests include physical disability and substance abuse, substance abuse among adolescents, and drug treatment evaluation. She has published in the areas of youthful offender treatment and correctional health care.

David Farabee is an associate research psychologist at the UCLA Drug Abuse Research Center. He is presently Research Director of a five-year evaluation of the California Substance Abuse Treatment Facility (funded by the California Department of Corrections), principal investigator for a multi-site evaluation of three residential substance abuse treatment facilities for youth offenders (funded by the California Youth Authority), and principal investigator for a study of substance abuse, medication adherence, and criminality among mentally ill parolees (funded by the National Institute of Justice). He has published in the areas of substance misuse, crime, and offender treatment.

This work was supported Office of Criminal Justice Planning Award No. RT96019501. The opinions expressed in this paper are those of the authors and do not necessarily represent the official positions or policies of the Office of Criminal Justice Planning or the California Department of the Youth Authority.

Address correspondence to Angela Hegamin, PhD, MSPH, School of Nursing, Health Science Program, California State University, Los Angeles, 5151 State University Drive, Los Angeles, CA 90032-8171 (E-mail: ahegami@calstatela.edu).

Treating Substance Abusers in Correctional Contexts: New Understandings, New Modalities. Pp. 139-162.
© 2003 by The Haworth Press, Inc. All rights reserved.
10.1300/J076v37n03_08

Predicting Retention of Drug Court Participants Using Event History Analysis

ELAINE M. WOLF

Center for Community Alternatives

KATHRYN A. SOWARDS

Center for Community Alternatives

DOUGLAS A. WOLF

Syracuse University

ABSTRACT This paper presents the results of a discrete-time event-history analysis of the relationships between client and program characteristics and the length and outcome of participation in a drug court program. We identify factors associated with both successful completion and premature termination. Having an African-American case manager, being older, having little criminal history, and not being a user of crack cocaine are strongly predictive of successfully completing the program. Predicted probabilities of successful completion ranged from 0.16, in the most pessimistic scenario, to 0.88 for the most optimistic scenario. *[Article copies available for a fee from The Haworth Document Delivery Service: 1-800-HAWORTH. E-mail address: <docdelivery@haworthpress.com> Website: <http://www.HaworthPress. com> © 2003 by The Haworth Press, Inc. All rights reserved.]*

KEYWORDS Drug courts, substance abuse treatment, treatment retention, case management, event history analysis, logistic regression

INTRODUCTION

This paper presents the results of an exploratory analysis of the relationships between client and program characteristics and the length and outcome of participation in a drug court program. Such programs provide an opportunity for nonviolent drug abusing defendants to obtain treatment under court supervision instead of serving time on probation, in local facilities, or in state prison. Our purpose is to examine how programmatic factors and client characteristics combine to predict success in the program. Programmatic features that relate negatively to success can, theoretically, be adjusted to improve program performance. Moreover, the ability to predict programmatic needs for special or intensive services for particular subgroups of program participants can help the court from a management perspective.

Although mandated treatment interventions have been shown to be cost-effective and successful at reducing drug use and harms in general, there remains a relatively high degree of failure for any given intervention (Anglin and Hser, 1990). Given that many defendants enter drug court as an alternative to incarceration, and thus have much at stake even beyond their recoveries, it would be particularly useful to know if certain participant characteristics are strongly predictive of poor outcomes. Depending on the charge, it is not inconceivable that opting for a relatively short incarceration term at the outset may ultimately turn out to be a more rational choice than drug court for some defendants in terms of criminal justice exposure. Some drug court participants undergo months of court supervision and frustrating treatment before failing or opting out of the program to face a criminal justice penalty. For some, the coercion and control of court-supervised drug treatment will ultimately be seen as a life-saving intervention, but for others it may simply be another extension of state control and interference in already troubled lives.

In this study we use survival analysis and data on clients' and program characteristics to identify factors associated with the outcome of participation in a drug court. Survival analysis allows us to compare long-term outcomes among different groups. With this model we are also able to retain explanatory information on all members of a participant cohort whether or not they had exited the program at the time of measurement (Hser, Anglin, and Liu, 1991).

BACKGROUND

Drug Treatment. Although many individuals, particularly those with strong social and material resources, manage to stop using drugs without formal treatment (Waldorf, Reinarman, and Murphy, 1992), addicts without those resources have been shown to benefit from treatment. Over the last 25 years numerous studies, including several national longitudinal outcomes studies, have led to broad-based consensus (at least in the public health field) that participation in drug treatment programs, whether voluntary or mandated by the state, reduces substance dependence and the harm caused by substance abuse (Leshner, 1999; Department of Health and Human Services, 2000). The four major national drug abuse treatment studies which undergird this consensus are the Drug Abuse and Reporting Program (DARP), which studied treatment participants between 1969-1972; the Treatment Outcome Prospective Study (TOPS), which studied participants in 1979-1981; the Drug Abuse Treatment Outcome Study (DATOS) conducted between 1991-1993; and the National Treatment Improvement Evaluation Study (NTIES), a five-year study begun in 1997 to evaluate the effectiveness of treatment for 5,000 clients in publicly-funded programs (Craddock, Rounds-Bryant, Flynn, and Hubbard, 1997; OJP, 2000). These studies involved tens of thousands of participants engaged in various treatment modalities across the country. All modalities demonstrated success in reducing substance use. A typical observation from the most recent NTIES study, for example, showed that treatment participants in federally-funded programs reduced their drug use by about 50 percent for as long as one year after leaving the treatment program. In spite of the general consensus, however, there is much to be understood about how and when treatment works. Not all types of treatment are effective for all people, and some individuals require numerous interventions, but studies generally show that all of the dominant program modalities are helpful for reducing drug use (Robert Wood Johnson Foundation [RWJF], 2001). As a result, drug treatment has been deemed "both effective and cost effective" (Institute of Medicine, 1996: 192).

An influential study in *The Lancet* (O'Brien and McClellan, 1996) has argued forcefully for a medicalized view of substance abuse, suggesting that it be understood much like any other chronic condition. It demonstrated empirically that treatment "success" for substance abuse was as high as or higher than that observed for such widespread chronic conditions as adult onset diabetes, asthma, and hypertension. As a consequence, they argued that it is unrealistic for an acute treatment to "cure" a chronic condition and asserted that relapse ought to be viewed as unsurprising, even expected, and not as a signal of failure. That view has been widely accepted (though not uncontested), and current thinking among many suggests that with multiple treatment episodes the clean time between use episodes lengthens and the duration of heavy use shortens gradually as exposure to treatment continues (Miller, 1999).

Several factors have been associated with success in treatment, including frequency and intensity of services, flexible and individualized treatment, and duration in treatment (RWJF, 2001), but methodological issues sometimes make it difficult clearly to understand the reasons for treatment's failure or success (Anglin and Hser, 1990). Magura, Nwakeze, and Demsky (1998) studied individuals who were admitted to 15 publicly-funded methadone maintenance clinics in New York City in order to identify pre-treatment and in-treatment predictors of retention. They identified three categories of in-treatment variables—problems encountered by patients, clinical responses to problems, and patient strengths demonstrated during treatment–and found that events during treatment are crucial for patient retention. The only pre-treatment characteristics that made a significant difference in the likelihood of retention were age (older people remained longer than younger ones) and involvement in the criminal justice system (those who had no involvement had longer lengths of stay than those who had previous involvement).

Duration of treatment has widely been shown to be associated with successful recovery or abstinence (Anglin and Hser, 1990), although it is unclear how much of this association is a result of unobserved heterogeneity among participants with regard to motivation. Wexler (1990), however, in a study of the impact of a prison Therapeutic Community on the likelihood of recidivism, provides evidence that clients who remain in treatment more than 12 months show shorter lengths of time until rearrest than do clients who complete the program in 12 months or less. Whether the Wexler findings were unique to that particular model and setting remains an intriguing question that is particularly relevant to research on drug courts, which typically subscribe to a minimum-of-one-year requirement for successful termination of their clients.

Drug Court Research. Research has also shown drug treatment to be effective for people involved in the criminal justice system, for reducing drug use as well as criminal activity (Anglin, 1988). Because of this, during the late 1980s and throughout the 1990s local courts began to re-think strategies for managing increasingly large caseloads of drug-dependent defendants and began to institute "drug courts" on a large scale. Although there is substantial variation in the implementation, administration, and outcomes observed for drug courts nationwide, they are generally regarded as promising models for reducing substance abuse (Belenko, 1998).

A growing body of research has focused on the ways in which drug court programs can be operated so as to minimize the likelihood of dropping out. Six recent studies focus on identifying pre-program and programmatic predictors of successful completion from drug courts, but they examine different populations, different predictor variables, and different ways of measuring similar predictor variables. Schiff and Terry (1997), analyzing the effect of participants' background characteristics on program completion, found that participants in the Broward County (Florida) Dedicated Drug Court Treatment Program were more likely to complete the program (graduate) if they were high school graduates, white, and not users of crack cocaine. A noteworthy aspect of their findings is that their model is better at predicting graduates than it is at predicting drop-outs.

In a study of the Escambia County (Florida) Drug Court, Peters, Haas, and Murrin (1999) used a Cox regression model to analyze the likelihood of program completion, focusing on clients' pre-program characteristics. They found that being employed full-time at the time of enrollment, being charged with drug possession, and using alcohol or marijuana rather than cocaine were significant predictors of graduation. The authors note the importance of considering the program's implementation stage in interpreting their findings: the court was young and in a state of some procedural inconsistencies as well as having few participants. Yet they argue that their findings suggest the importance of court administrators' paying more attention to risk identification and management (e.g., developing specialized supervision and aftercare programs) rather than risk avoidance.

Miller and Shutt (2001) propose that drug courts focus on stronger screening mechanisms in order to reduce failure rates. Based upon their examination of data from the Richland County (South Carolina) Drug Court, they concluded that having two or more prior convictions, crack use, being involved in criminal behavior prior to the onset of drug use, and prior drug treatment should disqualify a defendant from enrolling in that drug court program by virtue of their high failure rate.

Sechrest and Shicor's (2001) analysis is based upon their evaluation of the Riverside County (California) Drug Court Program. They found that the pre-program factors of being white, having the ability to be self-supporting, and not being a marijuana user were significantly associated with program completion. Their examination of variable programmatic factors was limited to the achievement of a GED or enrollment in college during program participation, which their data indicate significantly affects the likelihood of completion.

Senjo and Leip's (2001) study of the Broward County Drug Court is intended to test the ability of a model of therapeutic jurisprudence to predict successful completion of drug court requirements. They conceptualize this model as consisting of four components: court monitoring characteristics (captured as the judge's use of supportive comments during status hearings); treatment characteristics (captured as number of treatments of any kind); criminal procedure characteristics (measured as time between arrest and program enrollment, whether the participant was charged with a drug offense involving cocaine, and length of time in the program); and offender characteristics (age, race, education level, gender, marital status, and whether the participant was born in the United States). They found that the judge's use of supportive language and the participant's not having been arrested on a cocaine charge, being young, and being white were statistically significant predictors of program completion.

Finally, Rempel and Depies DeStefano (2001) analyzed many types of pre-program variables (level of legal coercion, demographic and socioeconomic characteristics, substance abuse history, criminal history, and neighborhood characteristics) and one type of programmatic variable (length of time between enrollment and initiation of treatment) using data from the Brooklyn Treatment Court and found that level of legal coercion, older age, and rapid initiation into treatment were strongly related to retention in treatment.

Belenko's (1998; 1999; 2001) reviews of drug court evaluations address the issue of retention and graduation rates. His earliest review of a few courts concludes that there is a relationship between the pre-programmatic factors of substantial substance abuse and criminal histories, but little prior treatment engagement, and client retention (1998). His more recent reviews of a larger number of courts indicate that courts differ fairly dramatically in the kinds of pre-programmatic factors that appear to affect the likelihood that individual clients will graduate. The data from eight evaluations that he reviewed most recently (2001), however, suggest that it is important to consider program maturity in predictive models. Multivariate models suggest that programmatic factors (e.g., imposition of sanctions and number of court appearances) are more important than individual-level factors in predicting retention and graduation.

CITY DRUG COURT

This study analyzes data from a drug court located in a mid-sized northeastern city. "City Drug Court" is a drug treatment intervention that conforms to the model of drug courts that has been promulgated and supported by the Drug Courts Program Office (U.S. Department of Justice) since the Violent Crime Control and Law Enforcement Act of 1994 (see National Association of Drug Court Professionals Drug Court Standards Committee, 1997). Three evidence-based assumptions regarding effective means of increasing the likelihood of recovery and reducing the likelihood of future criminal behavior underlie the design of most drug courts as well as the analysis we report in this paper: the importance of court-mandated treatment; the immediacy of treatment following arrest; and the "hammer" of facing a prison sentence.

The components of City Drug Court include offering a program of drug treatment in lieu of prosecution and adjudication to misdemeanor-level (carrying a maximum sentence of one year in a local facility) and felony-level (carrying a maximum sentence of at least four years in a state facility) nonviolent adults. The program entails scheduling regular and frequent courtroom appearances before the drug court judge for each enrollee; providing independent case management services through a community-based organization; enforcing a system of rewards and graduated sanctions as responses to participants' behavior; vacating the pleas and dismissing the charges of participants who graduate from the program; formally linking criminal justice and treatment agencies; and operating under a system of accountability whereby the court maintains an extensive monitoring system and complies with evaluation requirements. The program's design specifies that participants who remain in the program for a year or more, complete a course of drug treatment, and demonstrate that they are solidly into recovery by passing 12 urine screens are eligible to graduate.

The program is located within a court of limited jurisdiction and has been in operation since early 1997. As of April 30, 2001, 421 defendants had signed contracts with the court. Its typical caseload at any given time is approximately

100 people, and 56 percent of those who had left the program after a year or more were successful completers (graduates).

All drug courts want their defendants to succeed. Treatment providers, other social service agencies, case managers, and program personnel invest considerable time in assisting clients with obtaining Medicaid and other public assistance benefits; referring them to treatment services; providing treatment and other "wraparound" services; and monitoring clients' response to treatment. The goal of the court is to see a return on that investment in terms of sustained abstinence, engagement in productive activity, and avoidance of lawbreaking behavior on the part of its clients.

This research focuses on identifying patterns associated with successful as well as premature termination from the program. While the criteria for graduation are identified in its design, the judge has considerable discretion regarding the imposition of premature terminations from the program. The pathways by which drop-outs typically leave the court are of several types: an arrest for a serious offense; chronic relapse or abscondance from treatment; their decision that the court "just isn't for them"; and automatic expulsion for having an open bench warrant from the City Drug Court for six months or more.

Each participant in City Drug Court has a number of attributes, both pre-programmatic (e.g., age, race, and gender), over which the program has no control, and programmatic (e.g., case manager and treatment start date) over which the program does have control. We argue that identifying factors that can increase the likelihood of success will result in better outcomes for participants as well as greater efficiency and satisfaction for the court. Moreover, our methodological approach, which models the time-path of both successful and unsuccessful completion of the program, produces detailed forecasts useful for policy and planning purposes.

DATA AND METHODS

Data. Most of the data used in this paper were extracted from a database that was created and maintained by the first author for monitoring and evaluating the City Drug Court. This database consists of records of all persons enrolled in the court since its inception in 1997 through April 30, 2001, and contains information regarding participants' demographic characteristics, current charges, critical participation-related dates (arrest, enrollment, and initiation of treatment), drug of choice, and type of representation (Legal Aid or other). A second database maintained by the New York State Office of Court Administration provided several variables for the analysis (criminal history, current employment status, and educational attainment) that are not contained in the local database.

The dependent variable used in this analysis measures outcomes (*continue*, *prematurely terminate*, and *graduate*) for each participant for each month that he or she was enrolled in the court. The independent variables reflect participant characteristics and program characteristics. Participant attributes consist of demographic characteristics (male/female; African-American/European-American/Hispanic surname; age at enrollment), level of charge (felony/misdemeanor), employment status (employed/not employed), educational status (high school graduate or GED/not high school graduate or GED), responsibility for children age 18 or younger (living with children/not living with children), living arrangements (living with any other people/not living with any other people), primary drug (cocaine/other), and criminal history, as measured by convictions within the past five years and reported by the participant at intake (no misdemeanors/any misdemeanors; no felonies/any felonies). Program characteristics reflect the participant's form of legal representation (being assigned a Legal Aid attorney who maintained a consistent presence in the court/being assigned a non-Legal Aid attorney or retaining an attorney, both of whom are less familiar with this court's "culture" and procedures), duration of time between program events (between arrest and referral to the court; between referral to the court and contract signing; and between contract signing and initiation of treatment), whether the race of the participant's case manager matches that of the participant, and year of the court's operations (1997, 1998, 1999, or 2000-April 2001). Our multivariate analysis also includes several interactions between selected explanatory variables, such as the participant's and case manager's race, the participant's gender and familial/household situation, and past and current felony charges. All these interactions are suggested by findings from past research.

The universe for our analysis consists of the cohort of drug court participants enrolled from March 1997 through March 31, 2001 ($n = 397$). Since the source data track participation through April 30, 2001, all participants are followed for at least one month. From the original set, 11 cases were dropped because of missing data on selected explanatory variables. Substantial numbers of missing values existed for some variables contained in the state-administered management information system. For those variables, we recoded missing values to zero and added auxiliary dummy variables indicating that the respective information is missing. This "dummying out" approach to missing data produces estimates of covariate effects that implicitly condition on the fact that the variables' values are known, while the coefficient on the "missing value" dummy has no substantive interpretation.

Model Specification. Our goal is to identify factors associated with both successful completion of treatment, signaled by graduation from the program, and with failure to complete the program, signaled by termination prior to graduation. Furthermore, the time spent in the program by both those who have graduated and have been terminated to date exhibits considerable variation, and this variation may in turn be related to participant characteristics. We address all these issues using discrete-time event-history analysis techniques (Allison, 1984).

The key events defining a participant's history are the contract signing date, at which time a participant's program history begins, and the date of eligibility for graduation (if the participant is determined to have completed treatment successfully) or, for all other cases, of administrative termination from the program. As of April 20, 2001, 133 participants in our analysis cohort remained active in the program. These "right-censored" cases are, however, included in the analysis as explained below.

Although our data contain the exact calendar date of all relevant events, we have arranged our data in "person-month" format, with months measured from the date of contract signing. We have defined the unit of analysis as a month rather than a week or day for two reasons: the program's design anticipates participation for at least a year, and most participants who were dropped from the program were enrolled for three months or more (86 percent). Using months as the time unit provides sufficient detail to capture these features of participation patterns. Moreover, a finer time unit would not add to our substantive findings, while introducing considerable "noise." We included person-months spent in abscondance from the program as "active" time because, from the program's perspective, these participants were on the one hand still "alive" and had not yet definitively signaled that they either wanted to drop out or were otherwise ineligible to continue and on the other hand were nevertheless at risk of being administratively terminated.

In each month, either of two events can be recorded: either a participant is declared eligible to graduate, or is terminated from the program. If neither such event happens, however, the participant remains in the program for another month. Thus, for each participant i, and in each month t, we define a trichotomous dependent variable with categories *terminate*, *graduate*, and *continue*, corresponding to the three possible outcomes each month. We model the conditional probability of occurrence of the events *terminate* and *graduate*, plus the "non-event" *continue*, using multinomial logit. These are conditional probabilities (also known as discrete-time "hazards"), since they condition on the fact that the participant has remained in the program until month t. Each participant contributes to the estimation as many person-months as they spend in the program, from contract signing up to the month of graduation or termination, or, for those still active in the program as of April 20, 2001, up to the final month they are observed, at which point their event history is right-censored. Our explanatory variables consist of (1) a set of variables describing the participant's characteristics, criminal history, and experiences with the treatment court at the time of contract signing, and (2) a set of variables indicating the duration of participation as of month t. The model contains two sets of regression coefficients, as follows:

$$\ln\left(\frac{P[terminate_{it}]}{P[continue_{it}]}\right) = \beta_{10} + \beta_{11} X_i + \delta_{1t}$$

$$\ln(\frac{P[graduate_{it}]}{P[continue_{it}]}) = \beta_{20} + \beta_{21} X_i + \delta_{2t}$$

In these expressions X_i represents the (time-invariant) explanatory variables and δ_{jt} ($j = 1,2$) the effects of time in the program. We represent time using a set of single-month dummy variables through 18 months, plus an open-ended category for months 19 and higher.

Implications of Estimated Model. Using the estimated coefficients of our model we can derive a number of predictions. For example, using the notation $P[T_t]$, $P[G_t]$, and $P[C_t]$ to refer to the conditional probabilities of termination, graduation, and continuation, respectively, in month t, the probability that a participant will remain in the program from enrollment until month t–the probability of "surviving" up to t–is computed as

$$P[C_1] \times P[C_2] \times \ldots \times P[C_{t-1}]$$

The probability that the participant will survive up to month t-1, and then be dropped by the program in month t is given by

$$P[C_1] \times P[C_2] \times \ldots \times P[C_{t-1}] \times P[T_t]$$

while the probability of graduating in month t equals

$$P[C_1] \times P[C_2] \times \ldots \times P[C_{t-1}] \times P[G_t]$$

The preceding three expressions produce *unconditional* probabilities (in contrast to those embedded in the multinomial logit model), that is, the probability that a newly-enrolled participant will (say) remain in the program up to month t and then graduate in that month. There is an unconditional probability of termination (and of graduation) for each month $t = 1, 2, \ldots$, up to a maximum (which in our data is 38 months). Using these sequences of probabilities, the chances that a newly-enrolled participant will *ever* graduate (that is, will graduate in month 1 or month 2 or month 3 . . .) is given by

$$P[graduate_1] + P[graduate_2] + \ldots + P[graduate_{38}]$$

with an analogous expression for the probability that the participant will ever be terminated; these two probabilities sum to 1, inasmuch as one or the other outcome must happen eventually. Finally, it is straightforward to compute the expected number of months in the program overall, as well as the expected number of months leading to either termination or to graduation, using the sequences of unconditional probabilities described above.

RESULTS

Time Path of Exit from the Program. Figure 1 presents the monthly probabilities of the events *graduate* and *terminate* for months 1 through 29, after
which time the cell sizes become too small to permit meaningful calculations.
The lines trace out the "empirical" hazards, that is, the observed chances of
each type of event among participants remaining in the program in each successive month. Thus, for example, the probability of termination in month 1 is
about 1 percent, in month 2 about 4.6 percent, and so on. Figure 1 also plots the
survival probabilities, that is, the percentage of the initial cohort remaining active in each month. The survival probability is initially 100 percent, declining
thereafter; the median survival time–that is, the point at which half of the initial
cohort remains active–occurs at about 13 months.

The considerable irregularity in the time pattern of both termination and
graduation is no doubt due to randomness or to uncontrolled factors such as
seasonal effects or fluctuations in the court's caseload. In later months the increasingly large month-to-month fluctuations in event probabilities also re-

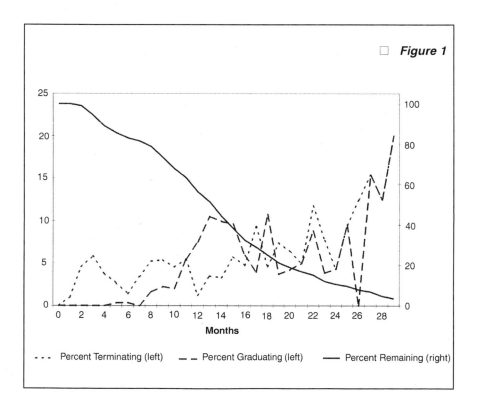

□ **Figure 1**

Months

- - - Percent Terminating (left)   – – Percent Graduating (left)   —— Percent Remaining (right)

flect smaller and smaller cell sizes. Apart from these irregularities, there seems to be no particular pattern of change over time in the probability of termination. However, graduation is rare at short intervals (one participant graduated in month five and one in month six), rising to a peak in month 13 and falling off somewhat thereafter. Our model is formulated such that the probability of graduating in months 1-4 is zero.

Multivariate Model of Program Exit. We present our multivariate results in three parts. First, we present and discuss the logistic regression coefficients. We then show the predicted change in each of the three monthly event probabilities associated with changes in the explanatory variables. Finally, we use the estimates to predict a hypothetical individual's entire history of program participation, month by month, and present several summary indicators of those predictions. We repeat the latter exercise for a range of hypothetical individuals that differ with respect to selected attributes.

Table 1 presents the average values of explanatory variables for the 386 participants included in our analysis, along with estimates of the parameters of our multinomial logit regression. As the column of means shows, most participants are males; are members of ethnic or racial minority groups; are not represented by a Legal Aid attorney; are charged with a misdemeanor; are not primarily users of crack cocaine (although participants who identify crack cocaine as their primary drug constitutes the largest group–41 percent–they do not constitute a majority of all participants); had not been convicted of a felony within the five years prior to intake; are not employed; had not graduated from high school or received a GED; and do not live with their own children but do live with other people. About half have a case manager that is of the same race, and half had been convicted of one or more misdemeanors within the past five years. On average, participants are about 31 years old, first appear in court about two months following arrest, took about one more month to sign a contract, and began treatment prior to contract signing.

As Table 1 indicates, most of our statistically significant results appear in the *terminate* equation. In particular, older participants are less prone to dropping out of the program. In any given month the odds of dropping out, relative to continuing, decrease with age. Similarly, people who report prior felony convictions have increased odds of termination, relative to continuation, in any given month. In the *graduate* equation, only the coefficient on the "crack" variable is significantly different from zero. The results indicate that participants whose drug of choice is crack have reduced odds of graduating, other things being equal.

The statistically significant race effects, which appear only in the *terminate* equation, are complicated due to the presence of an interaction between the participants' and their case managers' races. European-American participants have lower odds of terminating. Furthermore, when the participant and his or her case manager are members of the same racial group, the odds of terminating are also reduced (see the coefficient on "same race"). However, the coeffi-

☐ **Table 1: Mean Values; Coefficients of Event-History Regression**

	Mean[a]	Terminate[b] Coefficient	SE	Graduate[b] Coefficient	SE
Intercept		−2.8435	0.6005	−6.3022	1.0852
Female	0.39	−0.0128	0.3206	0.1810	0.4814
European-American	0.29	−1.2759	0.3367***	0.4479	0.3147
Hispanic	0.06	−0.3285	0.3736	0.6422	0.4279
Same Race	0.46	1.6929	0.3703***	−0.4140	0.4204
Same Race*Minority[c]	0.33	−2.4714	0.4409***	0.2034	0.5202
Legal Aid	0.18	0.0651	0.2204	−0.2789	0.3470
Age	30.7	−0.0341	0.0120**	0.0147	0.0161
Crack	0.43	−0.0226	0.2102	−0.8111	0.2677**
Felony	0.28	−0.2385	0.2418	−0.0371	0.3136
Past Felonies	0.26	0.7837	0.2563**	0.4090	0.3433
Felony*Past Felonies	0.08	−0.2017	0.4083	−0.9956	0.5564
Past Misdemeanors	0.51	0.2353	0.2489	0.1350	0.2895
Employed	0.17	−0.2187	0.2643	0.2079	0.3237
HS Grad	0.33	−0.2490	0.1936	0.3878	0.2557
With Children	0.13	−0.3427	0.4334	−0.3979	0.5392
Female*With Children	0.07	−0.2887	0.6266	−0.0443	0.7909
With Others	0.61	−0.1356	0.2986	−0.2660	0.4082
Female*With Others	0.19	−0.7566	0.3937	−0.0921	0.5540
Days to Court	63.5	−0.0014	0.0012	−0.0025	0.0018
Days to Contract	35.2	0.0023	0.0014	−0.0008	0.0022
Days to Treatment	−10.1	0.0005	0.0012	−0.0025	0.0018
Year 2	0.19	0.1563	0.2708	0.2152	0.3176
Year 3	0.30	0.1281	0.2787	−0.2404	0.3374
Years 4 & 5	0.34	0.6580	0.3243*	0.1071	0.5241

*$p < 0.05$; **$p < .01$; ***$p < 0.001$
[a] Mean in sample of 386 participants.
[b] Coefficients from multinomial logit with n = 11,079 person-month observations.
[c] "Minority" indicates participants categorized as either African-American or Hispanic.

cient on the interaction of "minority" (which indicates a participant is either African-American or has a Hispanic surname) and "same race" is negative and quite large, in fact large enough to more than counteract the main effects of these two variables. The implication from these results is that everyone does better with a minority-group case manager. The race interactions can be given a causal interpretation only if participants' and case managers' races are uncorrelated. To investigate this issue we computed the expected frequency of same-race case manager assignments under an assumption of random assignment: assignment is random if a participant is equally likely to be assigned to any of the case managers employed by the program on the day they enroll. We compared the expected to the observed numbers of same-race case manager assignments. Chi-square tests indicate that the null hypothesis (i.e., that assignment is random with respect to race) cannot be rejected for African-Americans and Hispanics ($\chi^2 = 0.132$ and 1.133, respectively, $df = 1$) but is rejected for European-Americans ($\chi^2 = 7.505$, $df = 1$, $p < 0.01$). More European-Americans have same-race case managers (47) than would be expected under random assignments (33.7).

The logistic regression coefficients in Table 1 are somewhat difficult to interpret, since they represent the change in the log-odds of termination (or of graduation) relative to continuation, in any given month. Moreover, in general, different values of each explanatory variable produce changes in *both* log-odds values, and therefore in all three monthly event probabilities. In order to illustrate the latter sorts of changes, we have computed the change in each monthly event probability associated with a change in each explanatory variable, other variables held constant. Table 2 presents these changes, focusing on the categorical explanatory variables. Because the model produces a probability for each event in each month, and those probabilities are different in every month, it is necessary to choose a particular month with which to illustrate these changes. We have chosen to use month 13, which is approximately the median length of participation overall. It is also necessary to pick a set of values for all explanatory variables; these are the values at which all other variables are held constant while each explanatory variable is, in turn, changed. We use the composite omitted category–that is, an African-American male, whose case manager is not African-American, is not represented by Legal Aid counsel, is not a crack user, is not charged with a felony, has no criminal history, is neither employed nor a high school graduate, has no children, is living alone, and enrolled during the first year of program operations–for this purpose. This configuration of values produces the baseline probabilities shown in the last line of the table. For each dummy variable used in the model, we then compute each probability when that variable equals one. The differences between probabilities in each case constitute our estimate of the partial effects of the explanatory variables on the outcome probabilities. Because the three outcome probabilities must sum to one, the three *changes* in probabilities must sum to zero. For example, notice that crack users have a termination probability just 0.003 higher than that of nonusers (in month 13), and a probability of graduating that is 0.067 lower than that of nonusers. Since in any month they can only terminate, graduate, or continue, the difference in continuation probabilities between crack users and nonusers is $0.064 = -(0.003 - 0.067)$. Table 2 also presents the changes in predicted probabilities in relative terms, that is as percentage changes from the baseline values. Thus the 0.067 change in graduation

☐ **Table 2: Partial Changes in Predicted Event Probabilites Associated with Changes in Explanatory Variables**

Effect of:	ΔP(cont)	ΔP(term)	ΔP(grad)	Continue	Terminate	Graduate
	Change in Probability			Percent Change in Probability		
Female = 1 (With Children = With Others = 0)	0.025	−0.026	0.000	3.1	−53.3	0.1
European-American = 1 (Same Race = 0)	0.129	−0.035	0.065	15.6	−73.1	50.8
Hispanic = 1 (Same Race = 0)	−0.076	−0.017	0.093	−9.2	−34.7	72.5
Same Race = 1 (Eu-Am = 1; Hispanic = 0)	−0.023	0.023	0.001	−2.8	47.4	0.5
Same Race = 1 (Eu-Am = 0; Hispanic = 0)	0.044	−0.025	−0.019	5.3	−51.7	−14.7
Same Race = 1 (Eu-Am = 0; Hispanic = 1)	−0.029	−0.033	0.062	−3.6	−68.1	48.5
Legal Aid = 1	0.024	0.005	−0.028	2.9	9.8	−22.2
Crack = 1	0.064	0.003	−0.067	7.8	5.4	−52.1
Felony = 1 (Past Felonies = 0)	0.012	−0.010	−0.003	1.5	−20.0	−2.2
Past Felonies = 1 (Felony = 0)	−0.089	0.046	0.044	−10.9	95.2	34.2
Past Felonies = 1 (Felony = 1)	0.034	0.022	−0.057	4.1	46.8	−44.2
Past Misdemeanors = 1	−0.025	0.011	0.014	−3.0	22.7	11.0
Employed = 1	−0.016	−0.010	0.026	−2.0	−21.2	20.7
HS Grad = 1	−0.039	−0.012	0.052	−4.8	−25.8	40.3
With Children = 1 (Female = 0)	0.049	−0.012	−0.037	5.9	−24.8	−28.9
With Children = 1 (Female = 1)	0.045	−0.021	−0.024	5.5	−44.6	−18.8
With Others = 1 (Female = 0)	0.031	−0.005	−0.026	3.7	−9.4	−20.5
With Others = 1 (Female = 1)	0.043	−0.028	−0.015	5.2	−57.4	−11.9
Year 2 = 1	−0.031	0.006	0.025	−3.7	12.5	19.4
Year 3 = 1	0.018	0.008	−0.025	2.1	16.1	−19.7
Years 4 & 5 = 1	−0.046	0.039	0.007	−5.6	82.3	5.1
Baseline Probability:[a]	0.824	0.048	0.128			

[a] Baseline probabilities refer to month 13 and are computed with all "Effect" variables set to 0.

probability for a crack user mentioned above represents a 52 percent reduction in the probability of graduating, other variables held constant. Finally, for variables that are interacted with each other, we show the predicted changes in probabilities for all possible combinations of the relevant variables.

The participant race effects shown in Table 2, given their interaction with the race of the case manager, vary substantially. Recall that African-Americans whose case managers are not African-American have monthly probabilities given by the "baseline" values. When an African-American participant is, however, assigned to a case manager of the same race, both the probability of termination and of graduation are considerably smaller [see the row for "Same Race = 1 (Eu-Am = 0, Hispanic = 0)"]. In other words, for African-American participants having an African-American case manager fosters retention in the program; whether it contributes to improved chances of ultimately graduating is addressed below. Both European-Americans with non-European-American case managers and Hispanics with same-race case managers do better, in the sense of having both higher graduation probabilities and lower termination probabilities, relative to the baseline case. European-American participants with a same-race case manager, however, seem to do worse: their graduation probabilities are no higher, but their termination probabilities are nearly 50 percent higher.

Predicted Patterns of Program Retention and Completion. Tables 1 and 2 presented our findings regarding the likelihoods of graduating, dropping out, and continuing in a given month. To make these findings more useful to practitioners and policy makers we have converted them to overall predictions based on different participant and program characteristics. We made comparisons based on variations in only those factors that were shown to have a significant effect on the probabilities of dropping out and graduating in Table 1: race, minority status of case manager, felony history, age, and crack as the primary drug. We also computed two composite hypothetical cases based on the values for these variables that would represent optimistic and pessimistic trajectories. Using the coefficients from Table 1 and the formulas introduced earlier, we computed a series of predicted values for the average duration of program participation overall, the probability of graduation, the average duration of program participation prior to dropping out among those who do not complete successfully, and the average duration of participation for those who ultimately graduate (because the sum of the ultimate probability of graduation and dropping out is 1, we chose not to report the probability of dropping out in this Table).

We first computed these values for a reference individual based generally on modal or average values for each variable. The reference individual represents predictions made for a 31-year-old African-American male who enrolled in year two, who has a case manager who was not African-American, whose attorney is not provided by Legal Aid, who is not charged with a felony, does not use crack as the primary drug, is unemployed, does not live alone, and has neither a high school diploma, a job, nor children. The reference individual has mean values for all other variables. Row 1 of Table 3 shows that the reference individual could expect to stay under supervision of the court for an average of 13 months. The ultimate probability of graduation was 0.44. Those who graduated were predicted to stay slightly longer, 14.7 months, compared to the predicted length of stay for one who terminated, 11.6 months. The subsequent rows in Table 3 illustrate the relative influence on each of these predicted values when the value of one of the variables has been changed in the prediction equation.

☐ **Table 3: Predicted Probabilities of Graduation and Average Durations of Participation**

Hypothetical Individual	Average Time in Program	Probability of Graduation	Average Time to Termination	Average Time to Graduation
(1) Ref. Individual[a]	13.0	0.44	11.6	14.7
(2) AA & Minority CM[b]	16.1	0.58	14.9	16.4
(3) Eur & Minority CM[b]	14.6	0.81	12.3	15.0
(4) Eur & Eur CM[b]	11.4	0.33	10.1	13.9
(5) History of Felonies	9.6	0.30	8.2	13.0
(6) Age = 21	12.0	0.32	10.8	14.3
(7) Age = 41	13.8	0.57	12.1	14.9
(8) Primary drug crack	14.5	0.27	13.9	15.9
(9) Low success[c]	12.1	0.16	11.6	14.7
(10) High success[d]	14.3	0.88	11.7	14.6

[a] Values for the reference individual: male, 31 years old, African-American, case manager not African-American, attorney not provided by Legal Aid, crack not the primary drug, not charged with a felony, not employed, not a high school graduate, lives with others, has no children, enrolls in year two, and has sample mean values for all other variables.
[b] AA = African-American, Eur = European-American, CM = case manager, Minority = African-American or Hispanic.
[c] European-American with European-American case managers, aged 21, felony history, and crack as primary drug.
[d] European-American with minority case manager, age 41, no criminal history, primary drug not crack.

For example, the second row reveals how changing only the status of the case manager to a minority status (leaving all other values equal to those in the reference individual) alters the predicted values. This shift increases the average program duration upward by approximately three months, increases the probability of graduation appreciably to .58, and increases slightly the program duration for all participants regardless of graduation status. Findings presented in rows 1 through 4 suggest that the interaction between participant's race and minority status of the case manager creates substantial variations, particularly when looking at the ultimate probability of graduation. This is relatively low, at .33, for European-American participants with European-American case managers; yet quite favorable, at .81, for European-American participants with case managers who are members of a minority group. Thus, having a case manager who is a member of a minority group increases the probability of graduation and extends the duration of program participation for both African-American and European-American participants.

Rows 5 through 8 allow for the comparison of effects for felony history, age, and crack use. Younger participants do not differ much (less than two months for any contrast) from older participants in terms of program duration, but the probability of graduation favors older participants, .32 vs. .57. A felony history predicts a relatively low probability of graduation but also is generally predictive of a shorter stay in the program, compared to the reference individual, for those who terminate as well as those who graduate. When compared with the reference individual, shifting only the primary drug of choice to crack, reduces the predicted probability of graduation by approximately 40 percent (.44 to .27) and increases the duration of participation slightly for all categories.

Finally, the last two rows in Table 3 reflect extreme case scenarios. Table footnotes c and d describe the characteristics of each hypothetical case. An individual with a cluster of variables, each of which would be predictive of a pessimistic trajectory, has an overall predicted graduation probability of only 0.16. On the other hand the optimistic cluster of characteristics suggests a very high graduation probability of 0.88.

DISCUSSION

Our findings are consistent with a number of prior studies regarding drug court retention. The significance of certain participant characteristics (race, age, criminal history, drug of choice, and living situation) and certain program characteristics (program maturity) in particular replicate other studies' findings regarding the likelihood of program completion (e.g., Schiff and Terry's [1997], Peters, Haas, and Murrin's [1999], and Miller and Shutt's [2001] findings regarding the negative effects of crack cocaine; Miller and Shutt's [2001] findings regarding the relationship between having criminal convictions and dropping out; and Rempel and DeStefano's [2001] findings regarding the negative effect of age and the positive effect of rapid initiation of treatment). Other variables of significance are inconsistent with other studies (e.g., Sechrest and Shicor's [2001] findings regarding the use of drugs other than marijuana being predictive of program completion and Senjo and Leip's [2001] findings regarding the positive effects of being young).

We found that some features of the program–race of case manager and the program's stage of maturity–were also linked to the average duration and probability of success among participants. Having a case manager of the same race seems to be relatively more helpful for non-white participants, and all participants have a higher probability of graduating when the case manager is non-white. How much of this effect is due to race, as opposed to the particular case managers reflected in this study, cannot be determined with these data.

The model suggests a relatively high probability of successful completion for older white participants whose drug of choice is not crack cocaine and who have been assigned to non-white case managers (0.792) but a very low probability of success for young non-white participants who use crack cocaine as their primary drug and who have been assigned to a white case manager.

Our model is unique in its inclusion of a case manager-related variable. We argue that this factor is critically important. City Drug Court case managers represent a personal link between the court and treatment. They provide personal services to participants (e.g., accompanying clients to appointments with public assistance workers) and are typically praised by participants during graduation ceremonies as being vitally instrumental in their recoveries. To eliminate them altogether from a model of retention would be to neglect one of the court's critical (and "fixable") components. Many other programs are based upon a case management model and would benefit from an analysis of this component. Indeed, as multi-site drug court studies are initiated in the future, they may find that offering case management services is associated with higher rates of retention, regardless of the particulars of the matching of clients and case managers (e.g., by race or gender).

We were surprised by the fact that a felony charge, even when interacted with felony history, was not a significant predictor of program outcome. Legal coercion has generally been shown to be a factor in the retention of patients receiving drug treatment (Satel, 2000), and recent work on identifying critical drug court outcome factors regards "leverage" (the weight of the penalty for dropping out) as significant (Longshore et al., 2001). Rempel and Depies DeStefano (2001) found that facing an incarcerative sentence was a strong predictor of engagement in treatment in the Brooklyn Drug Court, and Belenko (1998; 1999; 2001) has reported on the deterrent effect of this factor in his reviews of drug court evaluations. Currently, New York State law requires people convicted of a second felony to serve 5-15 years in state prison. Even if felony-level participants had never before been convicted of a felony at the time of their enrollment in drug court (which could possibly result in a sentence of probation), they or their attorneys should anticipate the consequences of having a felony conviction on a criminal record and regard that as a significant deterrent to dropping out of the program. Our data indicate that 38 percent of the participants who are charged with a felony report that they have been convicted of a felony in the past, although missing data make a definitive conclusion untrustworthy (24 percent of the participants had missing data for criminal history). Perhaps with official information (i.e., rap sheets), rather than self-reported criminal histories and more complete data, we could test the hypothesis that this has a deterrent effect.

An important but difficult issue in our analysis, as in other attempts to evaluate treatment courts, is the degree to which the effects of variables that measure treatment or procedural variations can be interpreted as causal effects. One of the variables shown to have significant effects in our analysis, "same race," falls into this category. However, our knowledge of the treatment court's procedures suggests the absence of systematic attempts to assign participants to case managers on the basis of either person's racial group. Furthermore, statistical analysis indicates that for two of the three racial groups distinguished in our model, African-Americans and Hispanics, the null hypothesis of independence between participants' and case managers' racial categories cannot be rejected. This apparent randomness failed to hold only for European-American participants. Thus for the majority of participants it seems reasonable to give the "same race" findings a causal interpretation, one with meaningful implications for program design. Nevertheless, there are a total of only seven case managers represented in the analysis (five minority and two European-American), and we cannot be certain that the "same race" effect holds in general, or whether it merely reflects unobserved characteristics of these particular case managers.

Our approach goes beyond those used in previous studies by virtue of its attention to time patterns as well as to program outcomes. For example, Peters, Haas, and Murrin (1999) use a Cox regression model to analyze retention in a Florida drug court program. While the Cox model can identify the effects of covariates on outcomes, it cannot produce predictions about the duration of participation. Our model produces both such predictions; indeed, our results show that some explanatory variables both lengthen duration and increase the probability of graduating, while others shorten the duration of participation while increasing the probability of success.

There are, nonetheless, many gaps remaining in our knowledge of the dynamics of drug court participation and of the factors associated with success. While all the drug court studies cited earlier include "pre-programmatic" (participant) characteristics in their models and most include at least one programmatic variable, little consistency exists in the ways that these variables are measured, except for the most concrete (e.g., gender and age). Because we find the Rempel and Depies DeStefano (2001) study to be the most comprehensive analysis to date, we have attempted to employ the types of variables they used and have included some variables from our state's management information system to achieve that goal. A fairly substantial number of cases in that database contain missing data in the variables we used, however, making it difficult for us to interpret their effects on retention. (This difficulty is apparently not uncommon: several drug court studies report that missing data presented problems in their analyses of this topic [Miller and Shutt, 2001; Senjo and Leip, 2001; Rempel and DeStefano, 2001].)

As of August 1, 2001, over 1,100 drug courts had been implemented or were being planned in every state (JPO, 2001). This large number represents a dramatic change for local court systems, substance-abusing defendants, and agencies that provide treatment and other related services. From the perspectives of management, advocacy, planning, and policy making, it is important to understand the impact of various factors on retention. To facilitate the analysis that will lead to that understanding it will be necessary for adult drug courts of all types (e.g., rural, suburban, and urban; pre-plea and post-plea; large and small; case-management-based and non-case-management-based) to devote considerable resources to the systematic collection of detailed information in electronic form. This is an activity to which many drug courts, pressed merely to keep up with reporting requirements, have assigned a low priority.

In an effort to provide some systematic comparative measures to the drug court community, the National Institute of Justice has funded the RAND Corporation to conduct a national evaluation of drug courts (Longshore et al., 2001). Although the researchers affiliated with this study have identified five critical dimensions ("leverage," or the weight of the penalty for dropping out; the seriousness of participants' histories in terms of criminal convictions and substance abuse; program intensity; predictability of the court's procedures, such as its response to a particular type of infraction; and emphasis on rehabilitation) that are predictive of graduating participants with a strong probability of maintaining sobriety and law-abiding behavior, their study is limited to a small number of courts and has discovered that most capture a very limited number of variables in electronic form, and that some have little more than a paper-and-pencil method of monitoring participants and activities (Turner, 2000).

The validity of outcome measurements is a second problem. In conducting this study we have discovered that many of the dates identified in the data for graduations and administrative terminations fail to reflect the court's "real" experiences with its participants. Because graduation dates are "artificial" in the sense that a group of people finish their participation on a date that is defined by the court four times a year, and not by a well-defined point in their recovery process, we examined case managers' notes in order to identify the date on which each graduate was eligible to graduate (defined by the court as three months following his or her finishing treatment) and found that most graduates (86 percent) finished treatment less than three months before their graduation date. Termination dates also fail to reflect the point at which participants effectively disengaged from the recovery process. Our examination of case notes revealed that 65 percent of the court's dropouts demonstrated no engagement in treatment during the 60-day period prior to their termination date. Indeed, 32 percent never demonstrated any engagement at all following their enrollment.

One hypothesis suggested by the finding that few graduates complete all official program requirements following their completion of treatment is that the court recognizes the desirability, from an administrative perspective, of letting go of certain currently abstinent participants in order to reduce the risk of holding indefinitely onto people who it may suspect are incapable of three months of perfect compliance. The court faces two choices when confronted with such "chronic stumblers" (Wolf and Colyer, 2001)–to wait for a period of abstinence and expeditiously graduate them or to wait for the next "slip" to terminate them. While our data cannot capture this dynamic, it is a critical component of the context in which the outcomes observed in this study take place.

Local and federal investments in drug courts since 1989 warrant strong research and evaluation designs to identify correlates of program success. Graduation ceremonies are inspiring but may signify little if courts are strapped for material and human resources, the members of their teams are not of one mind regarding appropriate responses to instances of noncompliance by participants, and they feel pressured to report successes even if it means stretching eligibility rules for graduation for certain participants.

REFERENCES

Allison, P.D. (1984). *Event history analysis: Regression for longitudinal event data.* Newbury Park, CA: Sage.

Anglin, M.D. (1988). The efficacy of civil commitment in treatment of narcotic addiction. *Journal of Drug Issues, 18,* 527-546.

Anglin, M.D. & Hser, Y.I. (1990). Treatment of drug abuse. In M. Tonry & J.Q. Wilson (Eds.), *Drugs and Crime, Crime and Justice: A Review of Research 13* (pp. 393-460). Chicago: University of Chicago Press.

Belenko, S. (1998). Research on drug courts: A critical review. *National Drug Court Institute Review, I*(1), 1-42.

Belenko, S. (1999). Research on drug courts: A critical review: 1999 update. *National Drug Court Institute Review, II*(2), 1-58.

Belenko, S. (2001). *Research on drug courts: A critical review: 2001 update.* New York: National Center on Addiction and Substance Abuse at Columbia University.

Craddock, G.S., Rounds-Bryant, J., Flynn, P.M., & Hubbard, R.L. (1997). Characteristics and pretreatment behaviors of clients entering drug abuse treatment: 1969-1993. *American Journal of Dug and Alcohol Abuse, 23*(1), 43-46.

Department of Health and Human Services. (2000). *Changing the conversation: Improving substance abuse treatment: The national treatment plan initiative.* Substance Abuse and Mental Health Services Administration, Center for Substance Abuse Treatment. November 2000. DHHS Publication No. (SMA) 00-3480.

Hser, Y-I, Anglin, M.D., & Liu, Y. (1991). A survival analysis of gender and ethnic difference in responsiveness to methadone maintenance treatment. *The International Journal of the Addictions, 25*(11A), 1295-1315.

Institute of Medicine. (1996). *Pathways of addiction.* Washington, DC: National Academy Press.

Justice Programs Office, School of Public Affairs, American University. (2001). All drug court activity by state and county (Aug. 01) (www.american.edu/academic. depts/spa/justice/).

Leshner, A.I. (1999). Science-based views of drug addiction and its treatment. *Journal of the American Medical Association, 282*(14), 1314-1319.

Longshore, D., Turner, S., Wenzel, S., Morral, A., Harrell, A., McBride, D., Deschenes, E., & Iguchi, M. (2001). Drug courts: A conceptual framework. *Journal of Drug Issues, 31*(1), 7-26.

Magura, S., Nwakeze, P.C., & Demsky, S. (1998). Pre- and in-treatment predictors of retention in methadone treatment using survival analysis. *Addiction, 93*(1), 51-60.

Miller, J.M., & Shutt, J.E. (2001). Considering the need for empirically grounded drug court screening mechanisms. *Journal of Drug Issues, 31*(1), 91-106.

Miller, W.R. (1999). *Enhancing motivation for change in substance abuse treatment.* U.S. Department of Health and Human Services, SAMHSA, CSAT.

National Association of Drug Court Professionals Drug Court Standards Committee. (1997 January). *Defining drug courts: The key components.* Washington, DC: Drug Courts Program Office, Office of Justice Programs, U.S. Department of Justice.

O'Brien, C.P. & McLellan, A.T. (1996). Myths about the treatment of addiction. *The Lancet, 347*(8996), 237-241.

Office of Justice Programs, U.S. Department of Justice. (2000). *Promising strategies to reduce substance abuse.* Washington, DC: Author.

Peters, R.H., Haas, A.L., & Murrin, M.R. (1999). Predictors of retention and arrest in drug courts. *National Drug Court Institute Review, II*(1), 33-60.

Rempel, M., & Depies DeStefano, C. (2001). Predictors of engagement in court-mandated treatment: Findings at the Brooklyn Treatment Court, 1996-2000. *Journal of Offender Rehabilitation, 33*(4), 87-124.

[RWJF] Robert Wood Johnson Foundation. (2001). *Substance abuse: The nation's number one health problem. Key indicators for policy, update, February 2001.* Princeton, NJ: Author.

Satel, S.L. (2000). Drug treatment: The case for coercion. *National Drug Court Institute Review, 3*(1), 1-56.

Schiff, M., & Terry, W.C. (1997). Predicting graduation from Broward County's Dedicated Drug Treatment Court. *The Justice System Journal, 19*(3), 291-310.

Sechrest, D.K., & Shicor, D. (2001). Determinants of graduation from a day treatment drug court in California: A Preliminary Study. *Journal of Drug Issues, 31*(1), 129-148.

Senjo, S.R., & Leip, L.A. (2001). Testing and developing theory in drug court: A four-part logit model to predict program completion. *Criminal Justice Policy Review, 12*(1), 66-87.

Turner, S. (2000). Drug courts: A national evaluation. Presentation made at the National Institute of Justice's Annual Conference on Criminal Justice Research and Evaluation. Washington, DC: July 16-19, 2000.

U.S. Department of Health and Human Services. (2000). *Improving substance abuse treatment: The national treatment plan initiative.* SAMHSA, Center for Substance Abuse Treatment.

Waldorf, D., Reinarman, C., & Murphy, S. (1992). *Cocaine changes: The experience of using and quitting.* Philadelphia: Temple University Press.

Wexler, H.K., Falkin, G.P., & Lipton, D.S. (1990). Outcome evaluation of a prison therapeutic community for substance abuse treatment. *Criminal Justice and Behavior, 17*(1), 71-92.

Wolf, E., & Colyer, C. (2001). Everyday hassles: Barriers to recovery in drug court. *Journal of Drug Issues, 31*(1), 233-258.

AUTHORS' NOTES

Elaine Wolf is Research Director at the Center for Community Alternatives in Syracuse, New York, and also holds a research appointment in the Sociology Department at Syracuse University. Her principal research interests are in program evaluation, criminal justice system processes, and chemical dependency.

Kathryn Sowards is Senior Research Associate at the Center for Community Alternatives and a former Robert Wood Johnson Foundation Scholar in Health Policy Research at the University of Michigan. She is currently studying treatment and recovery experiences among women mandated to drug treatment.

Douglas A. Wolf is Gerald B. Cramer Professor of Aging Studies at Syracuse University. His research centers on issues related to the living and care arrangements of the older disabled population, and on demographic and statistical methods.

The authors thank "City Drug Court" administration and staff who have generously shared information with the first author. The authors are also grateful to the New York State Office of Court Administration which allowed them to analyze a number of the data elements contained in its statewide drug court management information system and to the Drug Courts Program Office, U.S. Department of Justice (Grant # 97-DC-VX-0115) which provided the funds to collect the data used in this paper. The Sociology Department at Syracuse University provided an opportunity for the authors to present this paper at its November 2001 Writing Workshop whose attendees provided them with many helpful comments. The authors also received helpful comments from Marsha Weissman and Susan Adair of the Center for Community Alternatives. The authors assume full responsibility for the findings reported in this paper as well as for the conclusions they drew from them.

Address correspondence to Elaine Wolf, Center for Community Alternatives, Suite 300, 115 East Jefferson St., Syracuse, NY 13202.

Treating Substance Abusers in Correctional Contexts: New Understandings, New Modalities. Pp. 163-177.
© 2003 by The Haworth Press, Inc. All rights reserved.
10.1300/J076v37n03_09

Treating Substance Abuse Offenders in the Southwestern United States: A Report Evaluating the Long-Term Effectiveness of the Yuma County Adult Drug Court

SHERRI McCARTHY

Northern Arizona University-Yuma

THOMAS FRANKLIN WATERS

Northern Arizona University-Yuma

ABSTRACT This report summarizes data gathered from the 64 graduates of the Yuma County Drug Court from 1998 to 2001. Those who agreed to participate were interviewed at 3, 6, 12 and/or 18 months after graduation. Instruments used included the Addiction Severity Index, the CSAT GPRA Client Outcomes Measure for Discretionary Programs and a questionnaire developed to assess how well relapse prevention plans were followed. Rather than increased ELAPSED time from treatment, the variables that appeared to predict relapse were family problems, lack of social support and employment difficulty. ASI severity scales did not differ significantly over time for those studied, but the instrument did appear to be a useful tool in predicting relapse. The majority of graduates studied were able to successfully carry out their relapse prevention plans and graduation plans. Criminal involvement after graduation appeared to be significantly less than that of offenders who have not been treated in a drug court model and, for those who did recidivate, time to first arrest appeared to be longer for graduates than for non-graduates. *[Article copies available for a fee from The Haworth Document Delivery Service: 1-800-HAWORTH. E-mail address: <docdelivery@ haworthpress.com> Website: <http://www.HaworthPress.com> © 2003 by The Haworth Press, Inc. All rights reserved.]*

KEYWORDS Drug court, rehabilitation, cognitive behavioral treatment

According to a recent edition of the American Psychological Association *Monitor* (DeAngelis, 2001), psychologists have vastly underestimated the impact we can have in the area of substance abuse treatment. As rehabilitative measures such as drug courts are implemented by court systems internationally, this statement appears well founded. There is a need for trained substance abuse counselors who can work within the court system. This is an important area for forensic psychologists to familiarize themselves with, especially in rural areas. Drug courts are becoming increasingly common venues for dealing with those arrested for offenses related to substance abuse in the United States as they prove to be efficient, effective and less costly than incarceration. More than a decade has passed since the first drug court model in the U.S. was established. Dade County, Florida, implemented the model as a diversionary program for offenders facing charges of simple drug possession or use in 1989.

A drug court is a special court given the responsibility to handle cases involving drug-addicted offenders through an extensive supervision and treatment program. Drug court utilizes a case management team approach. The team is typically comprised of the presiding judge, the prosecutor, the defense counsel, a psychologist and/or substance abuse treatment specialist, a vocational counselor, a probation officer, education specialists and community leaders (Belenko, 1996). Drug courts are designed to motivate offenders to overcome their substance abuse problems and reconnect to the community as productive citizens, and to support them as they do so. In addition, these courts are intended to ensure consistency in judicial decision-making, enhance the coordination of community agencies and resources and increase the cost-effectiveness of sentencing and maintenance for those convicted of minor drug-related crimes.

Since the implementation of the first U.S. drug court, over 150,000 offenders have participated in or are currently involved with similar models. The current number of active drug courts in the U.S. exceeds 400, with over 220 more in various stages of implementation and development. More than 100,000 participants have graduated from drug court programs (Hora, Schma & Rosenthal, 1999; Robinson, 2001). Research on these programs suggests that 73% of the participants have retained and/or obtained suitable employment after completion of the program. Over 71% of participants complete programs, and this results in positive benefits to society that would not occur if offenders were incarcerated (Cooper, 1997). Over 750 drug-free babies have been born to drug court participants in the last decade. Over 3,500 participants have regained custody of their children and over 4,500 are again able to make child support payments (Belenko, 1998; Lewis, 1998; Peters, 1996, 1999). Recidivism appears to be lower for drug court participants than for those who receive other types of sentencing (Deschenes, Turner & Greenwood, 1995). The model appears to have many advantages from a social perspective, as well as from a cost-benefit perspective. It also appears to provide a useful arena for partnerships between psychologists and the courts (Foxhall, 2001).

A PSYCHOLOGICAL PERSPECTIVE ON DRUG COURT TREATMENT

Although many psychologists have often seen forced, or coerced, treatment as less than optimal, research suggests that, in the case of substance abuse offenders, there may be benefits. For example, beyond a 90-day threshold, treatment outcomes appear to improve in direct relationship to the time spent in treatment, with one year generally found to be the minimum effective duration for treatment (Simpson & Sells, 1983). Over 60% of those who enter treatment through drug court models are still in treatment after one year (Belenko, 1998) compared to only 10% of voluntary participants (Langenbacher, McCrady, Brick & Esterly, 1993). Clients who remain in treatment for extended periods of time apparently overcome much of the initial resistance coercion creates, as research on the outcomes of many U.S. drug courts shows successful outcomes despite initial perceptions of coercion on the part of participants, especially when continued individual and group counseling is mandated in the treatment program (Satel, 2001). Thus, from a psychological perspective, drug court models which keep clients in treatment with qualified clinicians for a duration of over one year, whether the initial entry is viewed as coerced or not, are likely to show success. Cognitive-behavioral therapy appears to be an especially useful approach with recovering addicts (Tiffany, 1990).

Assisting recovered addicts in dealing with cues to prevent relapse is also critical from a psychological perspective (Foxhall, 2001; Marlatt, 1985). Therefore, a drug court model that includes extensive focus on a relapse prevention plan is likely to assist in client success. Because "triggers," or people, places, things and events that have become associated with drug use through classical conditioning (Spurgeon, McCarthy & Waters, 1999), can also trigger relapse, long-term programs that establish new habits, social networks and living arrangements are likely to demonstrate more success. Goal-setting, and the increased self-efficacy and sense of personal control that arises from meeting goals are also likely to be important to treatment success. Certainly there is evidence that a variety of variables, including: (a) drug history, (b) history of physical or social abuse, (c) family of origin alcohol or substance abuse, (d) length of abstinence, (e) employment status, (f) social support system/access to services, (g) religious affiliation, and (h) cultural cohort variables related to age and ethnicity impact success rates. Type of treatment (group or individual; cognitive-behavioral or psychodynamic) and length of treatment are also related to success rates. Long-term individual therapy utilizing a cognitive-behavioral approach seems to show evidence of being the most efficient treatment strategy overall, especially when combined with goal-setting and social support which leads to improved self-efficacy. Education, job satisfaction, economic improvement, stable family relationships and friendships are also correlated with success. An effective drug court model should combine all of these forms of support for optimum success. Psychologists should have an important role in designing and delivering services for criminal justice agencies and courts that develop drug courts.

YUMA COUNTY DRUG COURT MODEL

County demographics. Yuma County, a rural area covering approximately 5,600 square miles in southwestern Arizona with a population of approximately 200,000 is located on the borders of Mexico and California. This area is considered the "drug corridor" by many U.S. justice agencies and use of heroin, methamphetamine and marijuana are reported to be especially high, proportionally, by those working in local criminal justice agencies. Yuma is a city of approximately 80,000. Several smaller communities, including Wellton, Mohave, Somerton, San Luis, Hyder and Rolle and two major military installations, the Marine Corps Air Station and the U.S. Army Proving Grounds, also are included in Yuma County. The economy is based primarily on agriculture, the military and tourism. Over 50% of the population are Latino or Hispanic. Other ethnic groups represented 2% Black or African American, 1% Asian, 1% Native American, and 44% White or Anglo.

Drug court history and mission. Yuma County's Office of Adult Probation and the Yuma County Superior Court began a drug court on March 26, 1998. Since that time, over 60 individuals have graduated from the program and approximately 60 more are currently involved. The mission of the Yuma County Drug Court is to counter the devastating effects of substance abuse on the community by providing selected nonviolent offenders with an opportunity to achieve a more positive (and legal) lifestyle. The program is voluntary. It includes regular court appearances before a designated judge, mandatory and regular drug testing, individual and group counseling, vocational and educational assessment, referrals for vocational training, education or job placement and group support. There are two tracks within the model. Defendants eligible for Track I are offered a choice between drug court participation and prosecution on pending charges. In Track II, previously convicted offenders on probation are referred to the court as a result of petitions to modify or revoke probation. Participants who successfully complete all requirements of the drug court are honored at a special graduation ceremony and have the charges against them dismissed (Track I) or probation terminated early (Track II).

Eligibility. In order to be eligible for the program, offenders must volunteer and must be legal U.S. residents, not currently on methadone treatment and with no current dual diagnoses. They cannot have any felony convictions for violent crimes or any pending or prior convictions for sex offenses, and they may not have any history of drug importation. Track I participants may have been arrested for possession of drugs or drug paraphernalia, use of drugs or low levels of possession for sale. Track II participants may have been convicted for possession of drugs or paraphernalia or other felonies in which it is determined that the original offense was related to a substance abuse problem. The offenses must be probation-eligible offenses, and the sentencing judge is given the responsibility of determining eligibility. Final determination of eligibility and acceptance is at the discretion of the Adult Drug Court team.

Treatment. Treatment is delivered in four phases. During the first phase of treatment, the focus is on stabilization, orientation and assessment of needs. This phase lasts approximately 8 weeks. During Phase I, participants are required to participate in group counseling sessions with a substance abuse treatment specialist at least twice weekly. In addition, one individual counseling session per week is provided and three weekly support group meetings (12-step or other approved recovery group) are required. Needs assessment, including psychological, social, economic and vocational summaries, is a focus of these sessions. In addition, a weekly court appearance, which is structured in a support-group format and weekly contact with the supervising case manager is required. Counseling is, thus, intensive and occurs daily. Breathalyzers are given before each group meeting and urinalysis is required, on an unannounced basis, three times per week. In order to remain in the program, no drugs or alcohol are allowed during this time, and assessed fees must also be kept current.

After successful completion, participants continue to Phase II. During this 22-week phase, a focus on intensive treatment and needs assessment continues. Twice weekly group counseling sessions continue. Individual counseling is reduced to once per month and support group meetings are reduced to twice weekly. One fellowship (faith-based) meeting per month is also required. Twice weekly breathalyzer testing continues. Drug testing is also reduced to twice weekly. Contact with the case manager and court appearances occur every two weeks. With the therapist, each participant develops a written draft of a relapse prevention plan during this time. Referrals for vocational/educational counseling to focus on designated areas for life improvement, such as life skills training, structured job search, General Equivalency Degree (GED) training for non-graduates of high school, vocational testing and job or career training are given and arranged. Financial/legal assessment and planning sessions which includes identification of outstanding legal matters such as warrants, tickets, child support and other debts and development of a plan to resolve these issues are also incorporated during this phase. As in the previous phase, in order to remain in the program, no drugs or alcohol are allowed during this time, and assessed fees must be kept current.

Phase three lasts for 10 weeks. During this time, group counseling is required once per week. Group support meetings are required twice per week and a fellowship meeting (faith-based) is required once per week. Individual counseling is discontinued. A mentor or sponsor from the support group or fellowship group is selected, and contact with this person must occur at least once per week. Breathalyzer and drug testing is reduced to once per week, on a random basis. Court appearances and contact with the case manager is required only once per month. During this phase, it is mandatory to have and maintain stable living arrangements, and to finalize and be able to explain the relapse prevention plan developed earlier with the therapist. Also, fees must be current and no evidence of drug or alcohol use may be evidenced.

The final phase lasts until graduation, and requires participation in one group counseling session each week, at least one support group meeting per week, drug testing and breathalyzer once per week, weekly contact with mentor or sponsor, monthly contact with case manager, monthly court appearance, monthly alumni meeting and participation in at least one organized recreational activity per month. In order to graduate, participants must have at least 120 consecutive days clean and sober, be showing consistent progress toward educational and/or vocational goals, be following their recovery/relapse plan successfully and making progress toward resolving any remaining legal problems. They must have successfully completed all four phases, make sure fees are paid in full and complete a graduation questionnaire.

Since 1998, over 250 cases have been referred to drug court. In 20% of the referrals, the client declined the option. Another 25% were declined entry for a variety of reasons. Of those who were accepted, approximately 50% graduated or are currently participating. The remainder were discharged for failure to comply with the requirements. This study examines the long-term success of a sample of graduates who successfully completed the program to assess the sustained effectiveness of this treatment option and recommends strategies for psychologists working to improve similar models.

METHOD

Subjects

All graduates (N = 64) of the Yuma County Drug Court were invited to participate in the study. Those who agreed (N = 29) were contacted by a trained graduate assistant from a counseling program following their graduation. Participants included 19 males and 10 females. Data was also available from counselors and arrest records on seven additional graduates. The remaining graduates refused to participate in the study (n = 7) or could not be located (n = 21). Thus, data is available on approximately 60% of the graduates.

Instrumentation

Each subject completed the Addiction Severity Index (Fureman, Parikh, Bragg & McClellan, 1996) and the Center for Substance Abuse Treatment Client Outcomes for Discretionary Programs Questionnaire (Substance Abuse & Mental Health Services Administration, 2001). In addition, subjects were questioned to see how successful they had been at following their relapse prevention plans. Additional interview questions determined the following:

1. Has the subject maintained a drug-free lifestyle since graduation?
2. Is the graduate gainfully employed?
3. Has there been future contact with the criminal justice system?
4. What steps have been taken to improve quality of life and how do graduates rate the quality of their life?
5. How do graduates rate the quality of their relationships with significant others?
6. Have relapses occurred? If so, what seemed to trigger these?

Procedure

Interviews were conducted by a trained graduate student from a counseling program at the convenience of the subjects. Subjects were contacted at intervals of 18, 12, 9, 6 and/or 3 months after graduation from drug court. A total of 40 interviews were conducted. Eight of the participants completed interviews at more than one data point. The interviews were administered either at the subject's home, workplace or another community location convenient to the subject. Each lasted approximately one hour. The research team then reviewed all interview notes and ASI scores and results were compiled.

RESULTS

Of the 19 males and 10 females interviewed, 4 males and 2 females reported that they had relapsed and were again using illegal substances. Although the ASI also screens for alcohol use, use of alcohol was not considered a relapse as it is not an illegal substance. Fourteen of the subjects, or approximately one-half, reported moderate alcohol use. Two of the subjects who self-reported drug relapse also reported alcohol use. Two more of the male subjects were considered to have relapsed based on interviewer observation and other reports. For purposes of this study, the seven subjects who have been re-arrested on drug charges or reported to be using by their counselors will also be considered to have relapsed. Thus, 15 of the 36 subjects on whom data is currently available have relapsed after graduating from drug court. Relevant information on each of the subjects appears in Table 1.

Details about each subject's drug history, length of abstinence, religious affiliation, history of emotional or physical abuse, history of family alcoholism, gender, age and ethnicity appear in Table 1. Interview data suggests that the focal questions can be answered, for this group, as follows:

1. Has the subject maintained a drug-free lifestyle since graduation? The majority of graduates have done so, but below the national average reported for similar programs.
2. Is the graduate gainfully employed? Although all but two graduates are currently employed, over half are in unstable, poorly paying and unrewarding jobs.
3. Has there been future contact with the criminal justice system? For five subjects.
4. What steps have been taken to improve quality of life and how do graduates rate the quality of their life? The majority of subjects report satisfaction. Two are continuing their education. Several more are making positive lifestyle changes, planning marriages or seeking career training or advancement. Material goals, such as vehicles or better housing, are cited by many and progress toward these goals is noted.
5. How do graduates rate the quality of their relationships with significant others? Thirteen of the subjects seem to have positive, stable relationships with friends and families. Limited social support seems to be a problem for over one-half of the group, however. This may be related to the unique problems of living in a rural, rather than an urban, area where fewer opportunities exist for establishing new social ties.
6. Have relapses occurred? If so, what seemed to trigger these, and what was the response? Over one-third of the subjects have relapsed since graduation. No clear patterns related to any of the variables examined seemed to characterize these relapses.

ASI Score Changes and Lifestyle Changes Across Time

Ten participants completed interviews at more than one data point. This data is discussed from a longitudinal perspective, below. Other interview results were compared from the perspectives of severity of ASI scores across time.

Summary of Changes Between 3 and 6 Months

Data was available on Subject Z at 3- and 6-month intervals after graduation from drug court. ASI interview ratings were zero on all dimensions at 3

☐ **Table 1: Drug History (DH), Length of Abstinence (LA), Religious Affiliation (RA), Abuse History (AH), Family of Origin History of Alcoholism (FA), Ethnicity (E), Gender (G) and Age (A) of Subjects in Yuma County Drug Court Study**

Ss	DH	LA (mos).	RA	AH	FA	E*	G	A (yrs.)
A	methamphetamine	36	Protestant	yes	yes	A	F	44
B	methamphetamine	36	None	yes	yes	A	F	43
C	opiates	--	Protestant	yes	no	H	M	49
D	opiates	--	Catholic	yes	yes	H	M	23
E	opiates	30	Protestant	yes	yes	A	M	40
F	methamphetamine	30	None	yes	yes	A	F	31
G	methamphetamine	30	None	no	yes	A	M	29
H	methamphetamine	30	None	yes	yes	A	M	20
I	methamphetamine	30	Catholic	no	yes	H	M	36
J	methamphetamine	30	Catholic	yes	yes	H	F	28
K	methamphetamine	30	Protestant	yes	yes	H	M	46
L	methamphetamine	30	Protestant	yes	yes	H	F	36
M	opiates	30	None	no	yes	NA	M	52
N	methamphetamine	30	Protestant	no	yes	H	M	45
O	methamphetamine	--	Protestant	yes	yes	A	F	35
P	methamphetamine	--	Protestant	no	no	H	M	27
Q	opiates	24	Catholic	no	yes	A	F	38
R	methamphetamine	24	Protestant	no	yes	A	M	30
S	methamphetamine	24	Catholic	yes	yes	H	F	31
T	methamphetamine	--	None	no	no	A	M	45
U	methamphetamine	--	None	no	no	H	M	30
V	methamphetamine	27	None	no	no	A	M	40
W	methamphetamine	24	Protestant	no	no	A	M	55
X	methamphetamine	24	None	no	yes	H	M	23
Y	methamphetamine	27	None	no	no	A	F	40
Z	methamphetamine	24	Catholic	no	no	H	M	40
AA	opiates	27	None	yes	no	A	F	37
BB	methamphetamine	30	None	yes	yes	A	M	20
CC	methamphetamine	24	None	yes	no	A	M	23

* A = Anglo; H = Hispanic; NA = Native American

months. At six months, a rating of 3 was assigned to "need for family counseling" and the subject reported difficulty with his girlfriend. He also reported health problems, and was receiving disability and unable to work. According to the data, he had not resumed the use of illegal substances at the conclusion of the study.

Summary of Changes Between 6 and 9 Months

Data was available on five subjects at 6- and 9-month data points. Subject N had ASI scores of zero in all areas at both interviews. He reported some health problems. He had secured steady employment in sales and reported rewarding relationships with his spouse and close friends. Subject P began using marijuana and amphetamines again between the 6- and 9-month interviews. At her first interview, she had been assigned a score of "2" on need for family counseling and a score of 1 on "need for employment counseling." At the second interview, she was assigned a score of 2 for "need for employment counseling" a score of 3 for treatment for drug counseling and a 4 for "need for family counseling." Custody problems, dissatisfaction with employment and unfulfilling relationships seemed to characterize her experiences during this time.

Subject V reported satisfying work and family relationships and planned to continue her education. She received scores of zero in all areas at both interviews and appeared to be functioning very well. Subject Y also received scores of zero in all areas at both interviews. She was not involved in a relationship, and was still living at home with her parents. She did not maintain her employment during the three-month interval, and was looking for work at the time of the second interview. She did report satisfying and supportive friendships. Subject AA was not working at either interview due to illness. He reported good relationships with his mother and children and no problems, other than health-related, were evident. He received scores of zero on all ASI dimensions at each interview.

Summary of Changes Between 9 and 12 Months

Longitudinal data was available at both 9- and 12-month data points for six subjects.

Subject I, who had an ASI score of zero on all scales except need for psychological treatment (score of 2), was arrested for theft and reported to again be abusing illegal drugs 12 months after graduating from drug court.

Notable changes during this three-month period for Subject J included leaving a girlfriend who was using drugs, becoming increasingly responsible for his children by a previous marriage and maintaining satisfying employment. ASI scores did not differ between the two interviews; all areas were zero at both interviews.

Subject K completed high school and developed stronger relationships with his children and family between 9- and 12-month interviews. His severity index scores were also zero on all dimensions at both interviews. He also maintained employment.

Subject L also received zeros on all ASI items at both interviews. She reported a supportive relationship with her husband, and was staying home to raise her three young children, one of whom is autistic.

Subject N reported health problems, increased responsibility and satisfaction at work and a supportive relationship with his spouse during the three-month interim between 9- and 12-month interviews. He also had scores of zero on all ASI dimensions.

Comparison of Self- and Administrative Report

Self-report data appeared to be reliable in most instances. In only two cases (subjects C and I) did there appear to be a discrepancy between administrative and self-report. This may be because of a self-selection factor, however. Graduates who were willing to participate in the study may have been more confidant of their ability to remain drug-free.

Comparison of ASI Scores Across Time

The ASI measures a client's need for treatment as perceived by the interviewer on a Likert-type scale of 0 (low) to 9 (high) in each of seven areas: medical services, employment counseling, alcohol problems, drug problems, legal services, family and/or social counseling and psychiatric and/or psychological counseling. As depicted in Table 2, most participants received scores of zero in all areas of the ASI. Means for each domain at each time period is presented. Each was assessed for significance at the .01 level via ANOVA. Although no areas were significant (likely due to the small sample size), several patterns were evident. Employment difficulties and problems with family and social support were most common. A qualitative analysis of the data indicated that these problems were generally precursors or co-occurring difficulties for those who did relapse. All of the subjects who relapsed had difficulties noted in one or both of these areas. Only two of the subjects who did not relapse had family or social support difficulties and none had difficulties maintaining employment.

DISCUSSION AND IMPLICATIONS

Life Domains Which Appear to Affect Substance Use Patterns

Longitudinal data suggests that maintaining strong, supportive relationships with family and friends, achieving goals and job satisfaction characterize those who succeed. When any of these factors are absent, subjects appear more likely to again begin abusing illegal substances. Long-term social support may be important for maintaining success. Employment counseling and support finding appropriate jobs also seems to be a necessary component to ensure long-term success.

ASI as a Predictor of Relapse

All subjects who relapsed except one had non-zero scores on the ASI in one or more areas. Family/social support were noted as problematic for nearly 60%

☐ **Table 2: Comparison of Mean ASI Scores of Yuma Drug Court Graduates in Each Domain at 3, 6, 9, 12 and 18 Months After Program Completion**

N =	3 mos. 2	6 mos. 14	9 mos. 9	12 mos. 12	18 mos. 3
Medical	0.00	0.21	0.00	0.00	0.00
Employment	0.00	0.07	0.22	0.50	0.00
Alcohol	0.00	0.00	0.00	0.00	0.00
Drugs	0.00	0.00	0.33	0.42	0.00
Legal	0.00	0.00	0.00	0.00	0.00
Family/Social	0.00	0.86	0.44	0.25	0.33
Psychological	0.00	0.21	0.00	0.58	1.33
Overall	0.00	1.36	1.00	1.75	1.67

Note: Range for each item is 0–9.

or those who relapsed. Employment was noted as an area of concern for 43% and psychological counseling was rated as a need for 30%. Of those who did not relapse, only 5% were noted as in need of family counseling and only 5% were noted as in need of psychological services. No other domains were rated above zero. Although the sample size is too small to justify quantitative analysis, these trends suggest that the ASI severity rating scale may be a valid predictor of potential for relapse and further study is warranted.

Fidelity of Relapse Prevention Plans

The participants, overall, appeared to be functioning well and not in need of treatment after their drug court rehabilitation. Their relapse prevention plans appeared to work effectively and they seemed able to maintain the skills they had acquired.

Among those who were not able to do so, social support and lack of rewarding employment seemed to be the most problematic areas. Several regional characteristics may make success particularly challenging. Establishing new networks of social support may be more difficult in rural than in urban settings.

Maintaining stable and rewarding employment in an economically disadvantaged region is more difficult. A long-term treatment model which focuses on enhancing social support structures with peers who do not evidence a history of substance abuse may useful. The Yuma Drug Court has responded to this need by initiating an "Alumni Group" that organizes social, recreational activities for graduates. This may help future graduates develop stronger positive social ties which are maintained after graduation. Training in areas such as goal-setting, time-management and career enhancement, as well as support for improved education, also seems warranted. Attaining goals is one of the most commonly cited reasons for life satisfaction by subjects interviewed. Long-term career counseling and job placement services also seem to be needed to enhance success of future graduates.

Criminal Involvement Between Graduates and Non-Graduates of Drug Court Compared

The success rate of Yuma County's Drug Court has been comparable to nationally reported drug court success rates which tend to be around 75%, and is above the greater than 50% recidivism rates generally reported for substance-abuse offenders who are not treated in a drug court model. Although local data on recidivism rates is not available in Yuma County due to a lack of funding (Valenzuela, 2001; White, 2001), observations seem to indicate a similar pattern (White, 2001). Despite the many regional characteristics which may make success particularly challenging, Yuma County Drug Court graduates appear to fare at least as well, and perhaps slightly better, than graduates of drug courts in other areas (Valenzuela, 2001).

CONCLUSIONS

This study provided important information about the precursors for success or failure of drug court graduates in Yuma County which may, perhaps, be generalized to others in similar rural areas. First, time did not appear to be a significant predictor of success or failure among the group studied. Relapse was as likely to occur at 3, 6, 9, 12 or 18 months after graduation. Rather than increased time from treatment, the variables that appeared to be important in predicting relapse were family problems, lack of social support and employment difficulty. ASI severity scales did not appear to differ significantly over time for those studied, but the instrument did appear to be a useful tool in predicting relapse.

This study supports the overall utility of incorporating a drug court model into rural criminal justice agencies to treat those convicted on drug-related charges. Not only is the model more cost-effective than incarceration, it is also better at preventing recidivism. The majority of graduates are able to successfully carry out their relapse prevention plans and graduation plans. Their criminal involvement after graduation appears to be significantly less than that of offenders who have not been treated in a drug court model and, for those who do recidivate, time to first arrest appears to be longer among drug court graduates than for non-graduates.

It is also worth noting that, for the group studied, self-report measures appeared to be reasonably valid. This finding needs to be interpreted cautiously due to the small sample size and the nature of the study. Use of volunteers, although required from an ethical human subjects standpoint, does likely introduce a self-selection bias among subjects.

REFERENCES

Belenko, S. (1996). *Comparative models of treatment delivery in drug courts.* Washington, D.C.: The Sentencing Project.

Belenko, S. (1998). Research on drug courts: A critical review. *National Drug Court Institute Review, 1,* 1, 1-42.

Carpenter, S. (2001). Cognition is central to drug addiction. *Monitor on Psychology, 36,* 6, 34-35. Washington, D.C.: American Psychological Association.

Cooper, C. (1997). *Drug court survey report: Executive summary.* Washington, D.C.: American University.

DeAngelis, T. (2001). Substance abuse treatment: An untapped opportunity. *Monitor on Psychology, 32,* 6, 24-25. Washington, D.C.: American Psychological Association.

Deschenes, E.P., Turner, S. and Greenwood, P.W. (1995). Drug court or probation? An experimental evaluation of Maricopa County's drug court. *Justice System Journal, 18,* 10, 55-73.

Foxhall, K. (2001). Preventing relapse. *Monitor on Psychology, 32,* 6, 46-47. Washington, D.C.: American Psychological Association.

Hora, P.F., Schma, W.G. and Rosenthal, T.A. (1999). Therapeutic jurisprudence and the drug court movement: Revolutionizing the criminal justice system's response to drug abuse and crime in America. *Notre Dame Law Review, 74,* 2.

Lewis, D.C. (1998). New studies find drug courts and drug treatment of prisoners, paroles and teens cut crime and drug use. *Physician Leadership on National Drug Policy,* 10.

Peters, R. (1996). Evaluating drug court programs: An overview of issues and alternative strategies. (http://gurukul.ucc.american.edu/justice/justb6.htm).

Peters, R. (1999). Current drug court evaluation results. Paper presented at the National Association of Drug Court Professionals 5th Annual Training Conference. Miami Beach, FL.

Satel, S. (2001). Drug treatment: The case for coercion. *National Drug Court Institute Review, III,* 1, 1-58.

Smith, D. (2001). Treatment for non-violent offenders: A wave of the future? *Monitor on Psychology, 32,* 6, 51. Washington, D.C.: American Psychological Association.

Robinson, K. (2001). Research update: Reports on recent drug court research. *National Drug Court Institute Review, III,* 1, 121-134.

Substance Abuse & Mental Health Services Administration (2001). Center for Substance Abuse Treatment Client Outcomes for Discretionary Programs Questionnaire. Washington, D.C.: SAMSA.

Turner, S., Greenwood, P., Fain, T. and Destines, E. (1999). Perceptions of drug court: How offenders view ease of program completion, strengths and weaknesses and the impact on their lives. *National Drug Court Institute Review, II*, 1, 66-85.

U.S. General Accounting Office (1997). *Drug courts: Overview of growth, characteristics and results.* Washington, D.C.: U.S. General Accounting Office.

Valenzuela, Y. (2001). Personal communication with director of Yuma County Drug Court program.

White, M. (2001). Personal communication with Yuma County District Attorney.

AUTHORS' NOTES

Sherri McCarthy, PhD, is an associate professor of Educational Psychology at Northern Arizona University-Yuma. She holds a doctorate in educational psychology with an emphasis in human development and cognition. She teaches courses in adolescent psychology, developing critical thinking skills, behavior management and personality adjustment. Her research focuses on teaching critical thinking and coping skills and on applications of psychology to education and criminal justice. She has written books on bereavement counseling and special education issues and recently had a chapter published on educational strategies to reduce the likelihood that adolescents will commit acts of terrorism in *The Psychology of Terrorism, Vol. 3* (Greenwood Press, 2002), edited by Chris Stout. Dr. McCarthy is active in APA's International Psychology Project through Division 2 and served on the organizing committee for the first international conference on the teaching of psychology for applied settings in St. Petersburg, Russia.

Thomas Franklin Waters, PhD, is an associate professor of Criminal Justice at Northern Arizona University-Yuma. He earned his doctorate in criminal justice from the University of Arizona with additional training from the University of Denver and the National Institute of Corrections. He has worked in rehabilitation programs in several prisons throughout the U.S. He recently completed a sabbatical project comparing opportunities for careers in criminal justice agencies for women in U.S. and Mexican agencies. Dr. Waters teaches courses in a variety of areas, including drug issues and the law, research methods in criminal justice and other current topics. He is active in the criminal justice community, cooperating with juvenile and adult probation agencies and police agencies throughout Arizona in a variety of projects and program evaluations.

This study was supported by the Yuma County Adult Probation Office and Northern Arizona University-Yuma. The authors would like to thank the Yuma County Adult Probation Department for their continued partnership and support conducting research on applications of psychology to prisoner rehabilitation. They would also like to extend their gratitude to Jenny Chong, PhD, of the Arizona Substance Abuse Consortium for Knowledge and Research. Sarah Kowalski, MEd, deserves recognition for the many hours she devoted to assisting with data collection for this project. Yolanda Valenzuela, Yuma County Drug Court Coordinator, and Judge Tom C. Cole, Presiding Judge, Yuma County Superior Court, deserve special thanks for their support and dedication to this effort.

Address correspondence to Dr. Sherri McCarthy, Department of Educational Psychology, Counseling & Human Relations, Northern Arizona University-Yuma, PO Box 6236, Yuma, AZ 85366 (E-mail: sherri.mccarthy@nau.edu).

Treating Substance Abusers in Correctional Contexts: New Understandings, New Modalities. Pp. 179-199.
© 2003 by The Haworth Press, Inc. All rights reserved.
10.1300/J076v37n03_10

Factors in Successful Relapse Prevention Among Hong Kong Drug Addicts

CHAU-KIU CHEUNG

City University of Hong Kong

TAK-YAN LEE

City University of Hong Kong

CHAK-MAN LEE

City University of Hong Kong

ABSTRACT This article reports on the findings of a study involving intensive interviews with 21 former drug addicts who had successfully maintained abstinence for periods ranging from one-and-a-half to four years. They were among the 74 successful former drug addicts out of a pool of more than 2,000 participating in a major rehabilitation program in Hong Kong in 1996. The intensive interviewing primarily employed a Q-sort task which required respondents to rate the importance of causes leading to their success in abstinence maintenance. The pool of causes was derived from ten theories that claim to explain drug abuse and recovery. Results show that the cognitive-developmental factor was the most important one followed by the social cognitive factor, which was significantly more important among former addicts who had maintained abstinence for longer time. These findings, therefore, uphold the particular relevance of cognitive factors to rehabilitation. *[Article copies available for a fee from The Haworth Document Delivery Service: 1-800-HAWORTH. E-mail address: <docdelivery@ haworthpress.com> Website: <http://www.HaworthPress.com> © 2003 by The Haworth Press, Inc. All rights reserved.]*

KEYWORDS Drug addiction, recovery relapse prevention, Hong Kong

INTRODUCTION

It is generally agreed that rehabilitation services for drug addicts have not been remarkably successful for a variety of reasons (Marlatt, 1985; Shiffman, 1987). First, few drug addicts join a treatment program voluntarily; second, a low proportion of those who join a program complete it; and third, up to 80% of those who complete a program have a relapse within a year. Hence, experience of the few successful cases is precious.

Drug treatment tends to achieve short-term success only rather than long-term abstinence and rehabilitation into normal community life (Ouimette, Finney, & Moos, 1997; Peters, Kearns, Murrin, Dolente, & May, 1993). Preventing relapse is, therefore, an important issue. Despite the plethora of theories on relapse, abstinence, and rehabilitation, research has not been able so far to identify causes of success and failure in the difficult process of long-term rehabilitation. For instance, biological causes such as detoxification and social integration such as social support and living with parents do not appear to be an effective predictor of successful rehabilitation (Bentler & Newcomb, 1992; Feigelman, 1990).

This lack of knowledge of causal factors has led most practitioners to adopt a multimode treatment approach. However, such amalgamation of treatment methods does not necessarily mean better results because it does not concentrate on effective causes of successful rehabilitation. It is also likely to miss causes that are effective (Beck, Wright, Newman, & Liese, 1993). Therefore, research that tries to identify causes of successful rehabilitation should adopt a long-term rather than short-term view in order to devise more effective treatment methods.

THEORETICAL FRAMEWORK

The theoretical framework of the present study draws on knowledge from two sets of social science theories. The first set of theories comprises social construction theory (Berger & Luckman, 1966) and its allies–ethnomethodology (Sharrock & Anderson, 1986) and symbolic interactionism (Hewlett, 1991). These theories stress the importance of human consciousness, reflexivity and understanding of the self and society in individual and social action. They presuppose that the individual cares about social phenomena, searches for patterns in them, becomes knowledgeable about the self and society and creates meaning of how they function.

These three theories represent the idealistic perspective in the social sciences which is different from the perspectives–the normative, the utilitarian and the power perspectives–which stress structural or cultural-traditional factors (Munch, 1987). The idealistic perspective maintains that the individual's self-generated thought–not conformity, calculation or ability–predisposes his or her action and satisfaction with an orderly world. In other words, common people can spontaneously construct theories to explain their life as well as social phenomena. These theories have been useful to investigate various social issues and problems in society: alcoholism (Sigelman, Gurstell, & Stewart, 1992); crime (Kuhn, 1991); homosexuality (Furnham & Taylor, 1990); poverty (Smith & Stone, 1989); illness (Furnham, 1994; Rogers, 1991); and drug use (Echabe, Guede, Guillen, & Garate, 1992). No study has yet used these idealistic, lay theories to examine abstinence maintenance from drugs.

The second set of theories comprises ten biological, psychological and sociological theories designed to explain drug abuse and recovery. First, biogenetic theory proposes that an individual's behavior is determined by his or her genes, hormones, other innate physical properties, and detoxification. Second, psychoanalytic theory, based on the biological theory, focuses on the inadequate resolution of conflicts generated by innate drives, particularly those of sex during childhood (Ellis, McInerney, DiGiuseppe, & Yearger, 1988; Leeds & Morgenstein, 1996). The result is an inadequate personality that predisposes the individual to drug abuse. Drug recovery depends on the individual's ability to overcome the unconscious conflict and to improve relations with significant others.

Third, social cognitive theory emphasizes simple learning as the cause of drug abuse and discounts the value of stable personality (Marlatt, 1985; Ouimette et al., 1997; Rotgers, 1996). The learning process can be both unintentional and intentional, and rational and irrational. Recovery, therefore, depends on whether the person believes in his or her ability to maintain abstinence and on whether he or she learns to appraise and cope with all problems associated with drug abstinence (Myers, Martin, Rohsenow, & Monti, 1996). Fourth, cognitive-developmental theory focuses on cognitive factors rather than faulty personality or social learning (Beck et al., 1993; Ellis et al., 1988). Personality is seen as the result rather than the cause of drug addiction. Fifth, rational choice theory posits that individuals behave in ways that maximize gain and minimize loss. Accordingly, one maintains abstinence only when it is easy and rewarding to do so.

Sixth, role theory assumes that the individual learns his or her roles in association with others (Helwitt, 1991). Each role involves a constellation of expected behaviour and can lead to social labelling. The label, "being a bad boy," can lead to the adoption of the role of a drug addict (Downs & Roses, 1991). On the other hand, the marital role tends to deter one's drug abuse (Burton, Johnson, Ritter, & Clayton, 1996). Recovery, therefore, depends on dealing with the social environment that creates the role and label. Seventh, social control theory that emphasizes the significance of the family, school, religion and other social agencies in society in both encouraging and discouraging the individual into and out of drug addiction (Gardner & Shoemaker, 1989; Umberson, 1987). Eighth, power theory is a version of the social control theory. The individual is forced into and out of drug dependency by strong agents (Hagan, 1988; Munch, 1987). In term of recovery, the police and other strong methods are seen as most important. Ninth, strain theory which stresses the individual's lack of identification with society as a result of, say, long-term unemployment (Agnew & White, 1992). This may lead individuals to adopt ways of behavior (including drug addiction) that they would not normally do. Recovery depends on dealing not only with the individual but also with the predisposing social factor. Tenth, consistency theory posits that behavior reflects one's attitudes, values, and other behavior (Munch, 1987). Accordingly, abstinence from drugs is consistent with the addict's orientation toward and practice of socially desirable behavior.

RESEARCH QUESTIONS

A list of 106 causes of drug abstinence emerges from the above ten theories. Although all of these causes are plausible, their absolute and relative significance are currently unknown. The study tries to answer two questions: (1) How do respondents rate the importance of these 106 causes and the related causal factors representing the ten theories for abstinence maintenance? (2) With increasing duration of abstinence maintenance, how does the importance of the causal factors become?

Both questions are contingent on the assumption that former drug addicts can be reflexive and conscious enough to articulate causal factors underlying their success in abstinence maintenance. Whereas the first question concerns the general importance of causal factors, the second question explores the importance as a function of time since abstinence. The foregoing review suggests that time can influence the importance of causal factors (Beck et al., 1993; Marlatt, 1985). It follows that identifying factors responsible for long and successful abstinence maintenance is of paramount importance.

METHODS

Data were based on interviews by one of the authors during April and May 1997 with 21 former male clients of a major non-government drug rehabilitation agency in Hong Kong. The agency offered a list of 74 male clients who had received treatment and who had successfully abstained from drug use for at least one-and-a-half years thereby closing their files in 1996. These 74 successful patients were a small proportion of 300 patients who completed the treatment project. Of the 74 successful clients, ten refused to take part in the study, 44 were out of contact because of change in residence or no response to invitation through mail, telephone, and paging service, and the remaining 21 were interviewed.

All 21 respondents had been heroin addicts and the vast majority had a criminal record related to drugs (see Table 1). Their average age at the time of the interview was 36.9 years (*SD* 12.5) while at the time of first drug use was 17.9 years (*SD* 3.7). They had maintained abstinence for an average period of 30.3 months (*SD* 10.4) and only two of them had occasional lapses.

The rehabilitation treatment offered by the agency included detoxification, rehabilitation in the treatment center and in the halfway house, vocational counseling, social work counseling and peer counseling. The treatment was a hybrid of various approaches and activities, including work and socializing.

☐ *Table 1: Distribution of Sociodemographic Characteristics*

	% (n)
Marital status	
Unmarried	66.7 (14)
Married	23.8 (5)
Cohabited	4.8 (1)
Divorced	4.8 (1)
Education	
No formal	4.8 (1)
Primary	28.6 (6)
Grade 7-9	42.9 (3)
Grade 10-11	19.0 (4)
Matriculation	4.8 (1)
Criminal record	
Drug-related	90.5 (19)
Others	4.8 (1)
No	4.8 (1)
Working	85.7 (18)
Counselor	27.8 (5)
Transport worker	16.7 (3)
Metal worker	5.6 (1)
Construction worker	11.1 (2)
Merchandizer	5.6 (1)
Mechanic	27.8 (5)
Warehouse worker	5.6 (1)

Intensive Interview

The intensive interview consisted of a Q-sort task and around 30 structured questions. The Q-sort task was a better method than direct rating for measuring the interviewee's attribution of abstinence maintenance. It required the interviewee to sort 106 cards representing causes informed by the ten theories (see Table 2) into ten piles on a continuum from (1) absolutely unimportant to (10) absolutely important, according to a fixed, normal distribution. The distribution was (1) 2, (2) 5, (3) 10, (4) 16, (5) 20, (6) 20, (7) 16, (8) 10, (9) 5, and (10) 2 cards. In the sorting task, the interviewee could easily reassign cards to different piles until he was satisfied with the output distribution.

The Q-sort is a method to enhance the quality of collected data. It especially matched principles of social construction theory that the individual can and does reflexibly construct meaning and knowledge for oneself to make sense of the world (Rogers, 1991; Senn, 1993). The theory criticizes the ordinary survey method with structured rating items for being too brief, artifactual, and unable to recover real meaning from respondents (Rogers, 1991). Hence, the Q-sort is also a humanist method which recognizes and extracts the individual's reflexivity because it centers on the subjective reasoning of the individual (Peritore, 1989; Rogers, 1991; Senn, 1993). The method is reputed for tapping the subject matter both extensively and intensively (Carlson & Williams, 1993; McKeown & Thomas, 1988; Peritore, 1989). Its intensive focus on the relative importance of causes is valuable for assessing self-referent and reflective causal attribution (McKeown & Thomas, 1988). The Q-sort essentially incorporates the individual's own analysis and interpretation necessary for making sophisticated decisions (Carlson & Williams, 1993; Rogers, 1991). To sum, the Q-sort encourages the individual to reconstruct causes leading to successful rehabilitation. In other words, the individual is to evaluate and compare the causes so as to compose a story about their relative importance. Because the concourse of cause items of the Q-sort had substantive theoretical grounds, it could reveal multiple perspectives on abstinence maintenance (Senn, 1993). The Q-sort effort could tap both the quality and quantity of causal attribution which neither open-ended questioning nor closed-ended rating could achieve (Rogers, 1991). Recently, the method has proven useful in revealing and testing theories regarding opinions on abortion (Werner, 1993), crime (Carlson & Williams, 1993), illness (Rogers, 1991), leftism (McKeown & Thomas, 1988; Peritore, 1989), pornography (Senn, 1993), and rebelliousness (Stenner & Marshall, 1995). Past studies using the Q-sort typically employed small samples and a size of 20 was common.

The biogenetic causes comprised those concerning detoxification, body structure, and dependence on drug to maintain health. The cognitive-developmental causes comprised those concerning intelligence, confidence, determination, knowledge, metacognition, rational thought, and moral development. The consistency causes comprised those concerning conformity to social

☐ **Table 2: Means, Standard Deviations, and Factor Loadings of All Items**

	M	SD	Loading on the respective factor	Maximum positive loading on other factors
Biogenetic cause (3 items, α = .426)	4.81	1.28		
My special body structure	3.62	1.96	.695	.316
My being not a precocious person	4.10	1.18	x	x
My having no need to depend on drugs to maintain health	5.24	1.73	.618	.482
My sex	3.43	1.36	x	x
My detoxification	5.57	1.91	.730	.356
Cognitive-developmental cause (8 items, α = .704)	6.49	0.88		
My wisdom, intelligence	4.86	2.33	.801	.185
My having confidence	7.95	1.69	.714	.193
My knowledge of the harm of drugs	7.43	1.29	.448	.297
My rational thought	6.52	1.25	.770	.218
My high moral development	4.62	1.50	.405	.248
My having determination	6.00	1.14	.463	.370
My belief in my method to maintain abstinence	7.00	1.34	.351	.127
My understanding of my thought and behavior	7.52	1.44	.556	.410
Consistency cause (5 items, α = .691)	5.89	0.97		
My dissent with drug taking	6.43	1.72	x	x
My dislike of drug taking	6.00	2.12	x	x
My friends' disapproval of drug taking	5.90	1.48	.598	.448
My will to maintain success in abstinence	7.38	1.24	.634	.154
My drinking no alcohol	3.52	1.69	x	x
My having no contact with old things	5.52	1.72	.672	.242
My maintaining abstinence in the past	4.52	1.81	x	x
My conformity to norms of society	5.38	1.36	.671	.336
Others thinking of me as able to maintain abstinence	5.24	1.41	.788	.205
Power cause (3 items, α = .528)	4.70	0.98		
My having no chance to contact drugs	5.05	1.69	.818	.309
None forcing me to take drugs	4.00	1.45	x	x
My being controlled by the police	3.05	1.56	x	x
My potential for maintaining abstinence	4.90	1.22	.632	.338
My having someone controlling my life	4.24	1.14	x	x
My being prohibited from contacting drugs	4.14	1.11	.704	.290
People of my occupation should not take drugs	5.90	1.95	x	x

	M	SD	Loading on the respective factor	Maximum positive loading on other factors
Psychoanalytic cause (11 items, α = .689)	5.37	0.79		
My not parading my superiority	6.19	1.50	.724	.124
My being controlled by parents and relatives	4.33	1.35	.598	.282
My being loved by the mother during my childhood	5.81	1.78	.660	.151
My not having a strong sexual desire	4.05	1.60	.345	.157
The harmony of my family	6.19	2.04	.514	.206
My family members having no distress	5.24	1.67	.531	.182
Parents' supervision during my childhood	4.48	1.69	.539	.303
My good temper	5.24	1.26	.488	.197
My control of emotions	7.33	1.49	.384	.315
My dislike of excitement	4.81	1.44	x	x
My having self-esteem	7.43	1.40	x	x
The stability of my emotions	6.00	1.73	.363	.280
My having no grievance toward society	5.48	1.72	x	x
My having no involvement in crime	4.14	1.62	x	x
My being abused during childhood	4.24	1.26	.291	.212
Rational choice cause (7 items, α = .655)	5.33	0.88		
My not having gone to the place at drug taking	6.43	2.11	x	x
Readiness to be caught by the police	3.90	1.51	.541	.414
Severe penalty	3.62	1.36	.537	.305
My ease of maintaining abstinence	4.62	1.47	x	x
Taking drugs benefits me nothing	7.00	1.64	x	x
My having no contact with syringes	4.05	1.40	.418	.348
My having no need to use drugs to lift my sexual potency	4.95	1.91	.683	.334
Maintaining abstinence giving me much benefit	7.71	1.68	.592	.417
My having no money to buy drugs	3.62	1.36	x	x
Many opportunities of my development	5.62	1.56	.623	.367
My having no place to take drugs	3.71	1.10	x	x
My having hope in my life	7.48	1.25	.591	.232
My desire for others' acceptance	5.67	1.49	x	x
My difficulty to get drugs	4.14	0.91	x	x

☐ *Table 2 (continued)*

	M	SD	Loading on the respective factor	Maximum positive loading on other factors
Role cause (5 items, α = .664)	5.47	1.32		
My need to be a good spouse	5.43	1.94	.795	.218
My need to be a good citizen	4.95	1.99	.454	.396
My need to be a good elder	6.43	1.47	.766	.380
My need to be a good offspring	6.33	1.65	x	x
My having a family of myself	5.29	2.26	.685	.119
My need to be a good parent	5.24	2.36	.637	.612
Social cognitive cause (10 items, α = .769)	5.94	0.88		
My acquaintance with people who maintain abstinence	6.67	1.65	x	x
My having no interaction with drug takers	6.81	1.60	x	x
No one persuading me to take drugs	5.00	1.81	.533	.340
My ability to cope with urges	6.48	1.54	.827	.433
My ability to confront withdrawal	5.33	1.53	.583	.495
My having ability to solve problems	6.33	1.59	.427	.432
My acquaintances' not taking drugs	5.43	1.86	.359	.228
My ability to maintain abstinence	5.95	1.69	.733	.365
My relatives' not taking drugs	5.19	1.40	x	x
My having skills to maintain abstinence	5.90	1.18	.491	.481
People whom I respect not taking drugs	4.57	1.96	.556	.193
My being convinced to take no more drugs	5.33	1.43	.514	.267
My good use of leisure time	6.71	1.52	x	x
My good use of money	5.33	1.98	x	x
My ability to cope with life stress	6.67	1.35	.514	.267
My self-control	7.00	1.48	.601	.194
Social control cause (14 items, α = .771)	5.52	0.82		
My need to exercise responsibility for society	5.33	1.53	.586	.331
My participation in activities in society	5.24	1.67	.543	.164
My having moral beliefs	5.14	1.62	.356	.291
Others' support	6.95	1.43	x	x
My belief in traditional values	4.29	1.55	x	x
My having a sense of responsibility for society	5.33	1.06	.512	.136
My belief in concepts that the mass in society endorses	5.57	0.93	.505	.410
My acquaintance with friends who do not take drugs	6.43	1.69	.553	.333
Others' expectation of me	6.86	1.96	.561	.244
My being controlled by others	4.24	1.41	.289	.260
Others' trust in me	6.95	1.63	.517	.459

	M	SD	Loading on the respective factor	Maximum positive loading on other factors
☐ **Table 2 (continued)**				
My family members' support	7.48	1.66	.283	.296
My intimate relationship with parents	6.00	1.64	x	x
My need to encounter the court	3.29	1.52	.618	.396
My faith in religion	4.14	1.93	.677	.256
My having a will to be a good person	6.76	1.87	.512	.238
Strain cause (8 items, α = .770)	5.41	1.06		
My having satisfaction with work	6.67	1.49	.667	.323
My smoking no cigarettes	3.67	1.93	.562	.348
My having income sources	4.62	1.77	.590	.292
My economic stability	5.71	1.87	.597	.373
My having a fulfilling life	7.19	1.63	x	x
My having a secure job	6.81	1.83	.660	.146
My having status	4.19	1.91	.644	.301
My having achievement	5.10	1.48	.612	.512
The timetabling of my life	5.81	1.75	x	x
My having ability to do things well	6.52	1.25	.703	.285

x: excluded from formation of the factor due to unacceptable convergent or discriminant validity

norms, past behavior, will, and friends' approval. The power cause comprised those concerning prohibition, potential, and chance of drug use. They reflected power or lack of power to use drugs. The psychoanalytic causes comprised those concerning attachment, parenting, sexual desire, and catharsis. The rational choice causes comprised those concerning the opportunity of development and contact, penalty, and sexual need. They reflected rewards and costs of drug abuse and abstinence. The role causes comprised those concerning roles of a spouse, citizen, and parent and having a family. The social cognitive causes comprised those concerning coping skills, modeling, and learning. The social control causes comprised those concerning responsibility, religious faith, and others' support and control. The strain causes comprised those concerning life satisfaction, well-being, and indicators of strain such as cigarette smoking.

Social integration was measured by a composite of sixteen 5-point Likert-type items. The reliability alpha of the measure was .861. The item-statements were: "I live with my family members in harmony at present"; "I have no sense of commitment to my current job (reversed scoring)"; "My current relationship to friends is in harmony"; "I dislike the present living environment (reversed scoring)"; "I know how to spend my leisure time"; "I am irresponsible for my family (reversed scoring)"; "I like the current job"; "I do not initiate interaction with friends acquainted during the time of drug addiction"; "I am satisfied with the current life"; "I am dissatisfied with the current relationship with friends (reversed scoring)"; "I am satisfied with the current family life"; "I am not satisfied with the current job (reversed scoring)"; "Some of my current friends are still addicted to drugs (reversed scoring)"; "I am not satisfied with the way of spending leisure time currently (reversed scoring)"; "I am satisfied with the current sex life"; and "I dislike current friends (reversed scoring)."

The usefulness of the treatment and rehabilitation was measured on a 5-point rating scale on six aspects, including the detoxification phase, rehabilitation phase in the treatment center, halfway house, vocational counseling, social work counseling, and peer counseling. The six items formed a composite score with a reliability alpha of .656.

The interviewee judged the helpfulness of the treatment to abstinence maintenance on a 5-point rating scale. For the ease of interpretation, scale values of all the ratings were transformed in the following manner: $1 = 0, 2 = 25, 3 = 50, 4 = 75,$ and $5 = 100$.

Analytic Strategy

To achieve a parsimonious causal representation of abstinence maintenance, two types of factor analysis, R-type and Q-type, reduced the 106 causes into a handful of factors. The R-type factor analysis used a multiple-factor approach (Gerbing, Ahadi, & Patton, 1987) to confirm the 10 theoretically based factors for the 106 causes. The multiple-group factor analysis approach employed correlations between composite scores and their constituents to confirm factor structure for a large number of items. It was especially useful when the number of cases was too small to warrant maximum likelihood estimation in confirmatory factor analysis via a LISREL-type algorithm (Anderson & Gerbing, 1988). The method would demonstrate convergent validity for composite score when it correlated strongly with its constituents. It would endorse discriminant validity when constituent items correlated more strongly with their own composite score than other composite scores (Cole, 1987). Another indication of discriminant validity would be weak correlations among the composite scores.

Q-type factor analysis analyzed the transposed data, with the interviewees forming the variables and causes as cases. The merit of the Q-analysis was its focus on interviewees and thereby their similarity and correlation with respect to a whole profile of causes (Rogers, 1991). It could then classify interviewees into factor-clusters. The resultant factors then best summarized the interviewees, not cause items. An underlying principle was for Q-type factor analysis to best reveal the self-referent subjectivity of individuals (McKeown & Thomas, 1988).

To assess effects of time on causal attribution, in terms of causal factors, stepwise regression analysis spotted significant predictors from a pool, including the duration of abstinence maintenance, social integration, family size, age at present, age at the first use of drugs, family size, employment status, and the criminal record. This procedure would minimize confounding due to other variables on effects of the duration of abstinence maintenance.

RESULTS

Multiple-group factor analysis confirmed the factor structure, convergent and discriminant validity of the ten groups of self-reflected causes of abstinence maintenance. The convergent validity was reflected by high loadings of items on their factors whereas the discriminant validity was demonstrated by the higher loadings on their own factors than the maximum positive loadings on any of other factors (see Table 2). For instance, the loading on the cause item "my special body structure" on the biogenetic factor was .695, which was higher than its maximum positive loading, .316, on another factor. The resultant factor structure that confirmed the theoretical framework, nevertheless, was a reduced one after having removed 32 items that failed to manifest either convergent or discriminant validity. Hence, cause items "my being not a precocious person" and "my sex," for instance, did not validly conform to the biogenetic factor. The remaining items could form reliable (α = .528-.771) composite scores, except the one (α = .426) of the biogenetic factor. The factors, the biogenetic cause and power cause that comprised few constituents were relatively low in reliability (.426 & .528). In general, these findings assured that the interviewees understood the causes in a theoretically reliable way.

Despite some significant correlations among the 10 factors of causes, no correlation was strong enough to indicate that the factors were identical (see Table 3). Furthermore, items loaded significantly on their constituent factors and less highly on other factors. This finding again upheld the convergent and discriminant validity of the factors at the molar composite score level.

The cognitive-developmental cause as a whole was the most important (M = 6.49, on a scale of 1-10, see Table 2) one perceived by former clients. Next came the social cognitive cause (M = 5.94). Cognitive factors were items considered as most important whereas the power and biogenetic causes were least important (M = 4.70 & 4.81).

☐ **Table 3: Correlations Among the 10 R-factors of Causes**

	(1)	(2)	(3)	(4)	(5)	(6)	(7)	(8)	(9)
(1) Biogenetic	1.000								
(2) Cognitive-developmental	−.030	1.000							
(3) Consistency	−.078	−.344	1.000						
(4) Power	.304	.232	.134	1.000					
(5) Psychoanalytic	.009	.065	−.030	−.097	1.000				
(6) Rational choice	.047	−.024	−.070	−.207	−.648*	1.000			
(7) Role cause	.262	−.368	.028	−.244	−.022	.129	1.000		
(8) Social cognitive	.200	.066	−.051	.468*	.049	−.295	−.078	1.000	
(9) Social control	−.601*	−.229	.403	−.082	−.416	.057	−.314	−.385	1.000
(10) Strain	−.036	−.065	−.522*	−.527*	−.166	.214	−.029	−.369	.074

*: $p < .05$ (2-tailed)

Focusing on interviewees rather than cause items, Q-factor analysis with the principal component method and scree test suggested that the interviewees clustered into four groups that accounted for 57.1% of variance. The first group, consisting of 8 interviewees (loadings > .450), showed high mean ratings and factor scores on items suggesting self-control (see Table 4). Interviewees of this group rated "my control of emotions" as the most important cause and "my need to encounter the court" as the least important cause. The second group of 4 interviewees (loadings > .556) showed high mean ratings and factor scores on items that were indicative of social support. According to this group, family members' support was most important and not smoking cigarettes was least important. The third group of 4 interviewees (loadings > .533) exhibited high mean ratings and factor scores on items reflective of self-efficacy. Confidence was the most important cause perceived by this group and not drinking alcohol was least important. The fourth group of 5 interviewees (loadings > .376) manifested high mean ratings and factor scores on items conveying life value. This group regarded having a fulfilling life as most important and special body structure as least important. Hence, self-control, social support, self-efficacy, and life values were four Q-factors reflecting the dominant causes of the abstinence maintenance of four groups of former clients, re-

☐ **Table 4: Means of Causes that (Positively and Negatively) Characterized the 4 Q-factors**

	Mean (Factor score)
Q-factor 1: Self-control	
My control of emotions	8.50 (2.33)
My understanding of my thought and behavior	8.38 (1.67)
Maintaining abstinence giving me much benefit	8.13 (1.84)
My having a secure job	7.75 (1.72)
My need to be a good parent	7.00 (2.34)
My economic stability	6.88 (1.73)
My good use of money	6.75 (1.95)
People whom I respect not taking drugs	*3.25 (−2.07)*
My faith in religion	*3.25 (−1.95)*
Readiness to be caught by the police	*2.88 (−1.77)*
My need to encounter the court	*2.38 (−1.97)*
Q-factor 2: Social support	
My family members' support	8.75 (2.40)
My acquaintance with people who maintain abstinence	8.75 (2.34)
My being loved by the mother during my childhood	8.00 (1.81)
My having no contact with old things	7.75 (1.70)
My wisdom, intelligence	*4.00 (−2.76)*
My having no contact with syringes	*4.00 (−1.72)*
My smoking no cigarettes	*2.50 (−1.96)*
Q-factor 3: Self-efficacy	
My having confidence	9.25 (3.01)
My ability to cope with urges	8.50 (2.16)
My will to maintain success in abstinence	8.50 (1.74)
My knowledge of the harm of drugs	7.75 (1.83)
My ability to confront withdrawal	7.00 (1.73)
The harmony of my family	*4.75 (−1.73)*
My being controlled by the police	*3.25 (−2.17)*
My having status	*2.75 (−2.09)*
My drinking no alcohol	*2.75 (−2.07)*
Q-factor 4: Life value	
My having a fulfilling life	8.60 (2.12)
My having hope in my life	8.20 (1.76)
My having self-esteem	8.00 (1.81)
Others' expectation of me	7.60 (2.27)
My having a will to be a good person	7.60 (1.92)
My having satisfaction with work	7.60 (1.83)
My acquaintance with friends who do not take drugs	7.00 (1.76)
My having achievement	6.80 (1.76)
My dislike of drug taking	6.60 (1.65)
My not having gone to the place at drug taking	*4.40 (−1.99)*
My having a family of myself	*4.40 (−1.76)*
My having no chance to contact drugs	*4.20 (−1.81)*
Parents' supervision during my childhood	*3.40 (−2.04)*
My special body structure	*2.20 (−2.19)*

spectively. Dummy variables were then created to identify membership in the four groups (Group 1 to Group 4).

As regards individual cause items, the interviewee regarded "my having confidence," a cognitive-developmental cause as the most important ($M =$ 7.95). In descending order, "maintaining abstinence giving me much benefit," "my understanding of my thought and behavior," "my family members' support," "my having hope in my life," "my having self-esteem," "my knowledge of the harm of drugs," "my will to maintain success in abstinence," "my control of emotions," and "my having a fulfilling life" all had mean ratings greater than 7. On the other hand, least important cause items were "my being controlled by the police," "my need to encounter the court," "my sex," "my drinking no alcohol," "my special body structure," "severe penalty," "my having no money to buy drugs," "my smoking no cigarette," "my having no place to take drugs," and "readiness to be caught by the police" ($M < 4$). Hence, whereas cognitive factors were most important, external power and control factors and noncognitive, biological factors were least important.

Besides, the treatment and rehabilitation services as a whole were helpful and useful for the former client's rehabilitation and abstinence maintenance ($M > 74$, on a scale of 0-100, see Table 5). The most useful ($M = 83.3$) service was that found in the halfway house while the usefulness of detoxification and peer counseling was relatively low ($M = 67.9$). The social integration of the former client was high ($M = 75.3$, on a scale of 0-100).

Regression analyses of causal factors with duration of abstinence maintenance, along with a set of predictors, were useful for testing the time effect on the importance of causal factors involved. Results indicated that one with a

□ **Table 5: Means and Standard Deviations of Social Integration and Usefulness**

	M	SD
Social integration	75.3	11.5
Helpfulness of treatment to abstinence maintenance	77.4	29.5
Usefulness of services	74.2	12.3
Detoxification phase	67.9	26.4
Rehabilitation phase in the center	82.1	14.0
Halfway house	83.3	16.5
Vocational counseling	63.1	24.5
Social work counseling	81.0	15.6
Peer counseling	67.9	21.1

longer period of abstinence perceived social cognitive ($\beta = .411$, see Table 6) or self-efficacy causes (.635), role causes (.215), and rational choice causes (.185) to be more important but perceived strain causes ($-.322$), social support causes ($-.220$), psychoanalytic causes ($-.187$), life value causes ($-.137$), and self-control causes ($-.117$) to be less important than one with a shorter period of abstinence. In particular, with increasing time, social cognitive or self-efficacy causes became significantly more important. Moreover, one who was employed perceived power causes as less important ($-.502$) than one who was unemployed. The police and authority appeared to be irrelevant to the employed person's abstinence maintenance. Social integration seemed to attenuate the importance of social cognitive ($-.569$) and self-efficacy causes ($-.417$).

DISCUSSION

Cognitive factors appeared to be the most important causes of success in abstinence maintenance as judged by former clients of a drug rehabilitation ser-

	☐ *Table 6: Standardized Regression Coefficients for Variables Predicting Causal Attributions*		
Dependent variable	Duration of maintenance	Employed	Social integration
Biogenetic cause	.024	-	-
Cognitive-developmental cause	.056	-	-
Consistency cause	.055	-	-
Power cause	−.058	−.502*	-
Psychoanalytic cause	−.187	-	-
Rational choice cause	.185	-	-
Role cause	.215	-	-
Social cognitive cause	.411*	-	−.569*
Social control cause	−.076	-	-
Strain cause	−.322	-	-
Group 1: Self-control	−.117	-	-
Group 2: Social support	−.220	-	-
Group 3: Self-efficacy	.635*	-	−.417*
Group 4: Life value	−.137	-	-
*: $p < .05$ (2-tailed)			

vice. They were especially important for those maintaining abstinence for a long time. Confidence, metacognition, knowledge, and rational thought were the most important cognitive self-reflected causes in line with cognitive-developmental theory, and self-control, coping ability, and problem-solving ability were the most significant skills conforming to social cognitive theory. Besides, self-control and self-efficacy were dominant themes emerging from Q-factor analysis. Taken together, cognitive-behavioral therapy should be the best theoretically guided and empirically relevant approach to maintaining abstinence. While many theorists and researchers have recommended the approach (Beck et al., 1993; Ellis et al., 1988; Marlatt, 1985; Rotgers, 1996), the present study is the first one to demonstrate the superior importance of its ingredients over other causal factors. It lends additional support to the empirical validity of the cognitive-behavioral approach (Rotgers, 1996). Compared with cognitive factors, biological, parenting, social norms, and control were less important. These findings support contentions against biological and psychoanalytic determinism in drug rehabilitation (Ellis et al., 1988; Marlatt, 1985). They suggest that abstinence maintenance and relapse prevention are long-term effort which requires favorable cognitive development and appropriate behavioral skills more than biological, intrapsychic, and social constraint. The latter, although relevant to achieving short-term success, may be inadequate to sustain long-term outcomes. The significance of cognitive factors is also in line with social constructionist (e.g., Rogers, 1991) and critical (Habermas, 1981) perspectives that presently attract much attention. They form the idealistic perspective discussed earlier in the article, which is independent of materialistic, utilitarian, and normative perspectives (Munch, 1987). This perspective holds that one's social construction, reflected by theorizing and understanding of social reality independently, contributes to the individual's well-being (Cheung, 1995, 1997).

With a longer duration of abstinence, social cognitive, role, and rational choice factors became more important and lack-of-strain, social support, psychoanalytic, life value, and self-control factors decayed in importance. These findings suggest that social cognitive, role, and rational choice factors might be especially responsible for maintaining abstinence for a long time whereas the other factors might be less likely to sustain the former addict's enduring abstinence. On the other hand, lack-of-strain, social support, psychoanalytic, life value, and self-control factors might be crucial for abstinence in the short run. They were, however, not likely to sustain abstinence in the long run. These inferences imply that long-term rehabilitation and relapse prevention programs should strengthen the client's social cognitive, role, and rational choice factors. This implication is consistent with the cognitive-behavioral approach that prevents relapse provoked by situational factors in the long process of abstinence maintenance (Marlatt, 1985).

The present finding is in favor of the cognitive perspective as an important explanation for relapse prevention. This favor is not supportive of the view that lapse is an automatic process which is noncognitive, fast, effortless, unintentional, and beyond one's awareness (Tiffany, 1990). Such a negative view, however, fails to adduce evidence to demonstrate both a sufficiently strong effect of the automatic process and an obviously weak effect of the cognitive process.

The importance of the social cognitive factor for abstinence maintenance tended to decline with greater social integration. This finding implies that social integration might substitute for one's social cognitive factor. In a broad sense, the substitution may reflect interplay between social integration as an external factor and social cognition as an internal factor. The salience of the external factor seemed to discount the importance of the internal factor. Such interplay might be a generalization of cognitive evaluation theory which states that the presence of external factors, such as reward, prevents an individual's causal attribution to internal factors (Deci & Ryan, 1985).

The present sample of 21 interviewees tended to be those really successfully recovering from drug addiction in Hong Kong. By using Q-method, the study may best unfold the self-referent subjectivity of former addicts when Q-method gears to the importance of studying a few persons intensively (McKeown & Thomas, 1988). Accordingly, it is valuable to investigate a few persons according to their self-referent, subjective frame of reference rather than a large number of people with an imposed frame. The approach maintains that scientific inquiry requires intensive analysis of structure, no matter whether it is objective or subjective. However, the findings may not be generalizable to drug addicts whose rehabilitation is not successful. At least, several thousands of drug addicts join the treatment program each year. Using the present approach to investigate these people should offer great value for their rehabilitation. Further, the study can employ a prospective design to adequately assess and monitor effects due to treatment and various causal factors. The design should offer much prognostic value for drug rehabilitation.

Although the sample was small, it might be useful for describing and making inference about drug addicts who had successfully maintained abstinence for a period longer than one-and-a-half years. Nevertheless, the successfully rehabilitated drug addicts are likely to be substantially different from the unsuccessful ones. Generalization of the present findings to the unsuccessful people may not be appropriate.

More data collected from diverse societies and cultures are certainly desirable. Besides corroborating present findings, they can facilitate multilevel analysis which treats the sociocultural context as a random factor and its effects in turn are contingent on factors at the sociocultural level. Such analysis is necessary for examining any cultural bias due to the context of Hong Kong that is responsible for present findings. The society and culture of Hong Kong are peculiar and unlike their Chinese origin. They are somewhere in the middle between Chinese and Western forms. Answers to the question regarding whether the findings are idiosyncratic can only be available from analysis of cross-cultural data.

The present findings support that rehabilitation services are most effective if they make use of the cognitive-behavioral approach. The cognitive emphasis of the approach should strengthen the client's confidence, understanding of own thought and behavior, knowledge of the harm of drugs, rational thought, including a realistic appraisal of situations, and determination (Ellis et al., 1988; Marlatt, 1985; Myers et al., 1996). Regarding behavioral empowerment, the approach should enhance the client's self-control, ability to cope with life stress, ability to cope with urges, and ability to solve problems. The approach can apply techniques used for rational-emotive therapy (Ellis et al., 1988) and cognitive therapy (Beck et al., 1993). Despite all this, rehabilitation services should not neglect social support and life value which are also dominant causes of the abstinence maintenance of some clients. The findings are supportive of applying the cognitive-behavioral approach in rehabilitation services.

REFERENCES

Agnew, R., & White, H.R. (1992). An empirical test of general strain theory. *Criminology, 30*, 475-499.

Anderson, J.C., & Gerbing, D.W. (1988). Structural equation modeling in practice: A review and recommended two-step approach. *Psychological Bulletin, 103*, 411-423.

Beck, A.T., Wright, F.D., Newman, C.F., & Liese, B.S. (1993). *Cognitive therapy of substance abuse.* New York: Guilford.

Bentler, P.M., & Newcomb, M.D. (1992). Linear structural equation modeling with nonnormal continous variables applications: Relations among social support, drug use, and health in young adults. In J.H. Dwyer, M. Feinleib, P. Lippert & H. Hoffmeister (Eds.), *Statistical models for longitudinal studies of health* (pp. 132-160). New York: Oxford University Press.

Berger, P.L., & Luckmann, T. (1966). *The social construction of reality.* London. Penguin.

Burton, R.P.D., Johnson, R.J., Ritter, C., & Clayton, R.R. (1996). The effects of role socialization on the initiation of cocaine use: An event history analysis for adolescence into middle adulthood. *Journal of Health and Social Behavior, 37*, 75-90.

Carlson, J.M., & Williams, T. (1993). Perspectives on the seriousness of crimes. *Social Science Research, 22*, 190-207.

Cheung, C.K. (1995). Political theorizing and well-being. *Journal of Social Behavior and Personality, 10*, 609-630.

Cheung, C.K. (1997). World understanding and well-being in a marital context. *Journal of Genetic Psychology, 158*, 41-58.

Cole, D.A. (1987). Utility of confirmatory factor analysis in test validation research. *Journal of Consulting and Clinical Psychology, 55*, 584-594.

Deci, E.L., & Ryan, R.M. (1985). *Intrinsic motivation and self-determination in human behavior.* New York: Plenum Press.

Downs, W.R., & Rose, S.R. (1991). The relationship of adolescent peer groups to the incidence of psychosocial problems. *Adolescence, 20,* 473-492.

Echabe, A.E., Guede, E.F., Guillen, C.S., & Garate, J.F.V. (1992). Social representations of drugs, causal judgment and social perception. *European Journal of Social Psychology, 22,* 73-84.

Ellis, A., McInerney, J.F., DiGiuseppe, R., & Yearger, R.J. (1988). *Rational-emotive therapy with alcoholics and substance abusers.* Boston, MA: Allyn & Bacon.

Feigelman, W. (1990). *Treating teenage drug abuse in day care setting.* New York: Praeger.

Furnham, A. (1988). *Lay theories: Everyday understanding of problems in the social sciences.* Oxford, England: Pergamon Press.

Furnham, A., & Taylor, L. (1990). Lay theories of homosexuality: Aetiology, behaviors and cures. *British Journal of Social Psychology, 29,* 135-147.

Furnham, A. (1994). Explaining health and others' lay perceptions on current and future health: The causes of illness and the nature of recovery. *Social Science and Medicine, 39,* 715-725.

Gardner, L., & Shoemaker, D.L. (1989). Social bonding and delinquency: A comparative analysis. *Sociological Quarterly, 30,* 481-500.

Gerbing, D.W., Ahadi, S.A., & Patton, J.H. (1987). Toward a conceptualization of impulsivity: Components across the behavioral and self-report domains. *Multivariate Behavioral Research, 22,* 357-379.

Habermas, J. (1981). *The theory of communicative action* (Vol. 1 & 2). Cambridge: Polity Press.

Hagan, J. (1988). *Structural criminology.* Cambridge: Polity.

Heiss, J. (1981). Social roles. In M. Rosenberg & R.H. Turner (Eds.), *Social psychology: Sociological perspectives* (pp. 94-129). New York: Basic Books.

Hewitt, J.P. (1991). *Self and society: A symbolic interactionist social psychology.* Boston, MA: Allyn and Bacon.

Kuhn, D. (1991). *The skills of argument.* Cambridge: Cambridge University Press.

Leeds, J., & Morgenstein, J. (1996). Psychoanalytic theories of substance abuse. In F. Rotgers, D.S. Keller & J. Morgenstein (Eds.), *Treating substance abuse: Theory and technique* (pp. 68-83). New York: Guilford.

Marlatt, G.A. (1985). *Relapse prevention: Maintenance strategies in the treatment of addictive behaviors.* New York: Guilford.

McKeown, B., & Thomas, D. (1988). *Q methodology.* Newbury Park, CA: Sage.

Munch, R. (1987). *Theory of action: Towards a new synthesis going beyond Parsons.* London: Routledge & Kegan Paul.

Myers, M.G., Martin, R.A, Rohsenow, D.J., & Monti, P.M. (1996). The relapse situation appraisal questionnaire: Initial psychometric characteristics and validation. *Psychology of Addictive Behaviors, 10,* 237-247.

Ouimette, P.C., Finney, J.W., & Moos, R.H. (1997). Twelve-step and cognitive-behavioral treatment for substance abuse: A comparison of treatment effectiveness. *Journal of Consulting and Clinical Psychology, 65,* 230-240.

Peritore, N.P. (1989). Brazilian party left opinion: A Q-methodology profile. *Political Psychology, 10,* 675-702.

Peters, R.H., Kearns, W.D., Murrin, M.R., Dolente, A.S., & May, R.L., II. (1993). Examining the effectiveness of in-jail substance abuse treatment. *Journal of Offender Rehabilitation, 19*(3/4), 1-39.

Rogers, W.S. (1991). *Explaining health and illness: An exploration of diversity.* New York: Harvester Wheatsheaf.

Rotgers, F. (1996). Behavioral theory of substance abuse treatment: Bringing science to bear on practice. In F. Rotgers, D.S. Keller & J. Morgenstein (Eds.), *Treating substance abuse: Theory and technique* (pp. 174-240). New York: Guilford.

Senn, C.Y. (1993). Women's multiple perspectives and experiences with pornography. *Psychology of Women Quarterly, 17,* 319-341.

Sharrock, W., & Anderson, B. (1986). *The ethnomethodologists.* Chichester, England: Ellis Horwood.

Shiffman, S. (1987). Maintenance and relapse coping with temptation. In T.D. Nirenberg & S.A. Maisto (Eds.), *Developments in the assessment and treatment of addictive behaviors* (pp. 353-385). Norwood, NJ: Ablex.

Sigelman, C.K., Gurstell, S.A., & Stewart, A.K. (1992). The development of lay theories of problem drinking: Causes and cures. *Journal of Adolescent Research, 7,* 292-312.

Smith, K., & Stone, L.H. (1989). Rags, riches, and bootstraps: Beliefs about the causes of wealth and poverty. *Sociological Quarterly, 30,* 93-107.

Stenner, P., & Marshall, H. (1995). A Q methodological study of rebelliousness. *European Journal of Social Psychology, 25,* 621-636.

Tiffany, S.T. (1990). A cognitive model of drug users and drug use behavior: Role of automatic and nonautomatic processes. *Psychological Review, 97,* 147-168.

Umberson, D. (1987). Family status and health behaviors: Social control as a dimension of social integration. *Journal of Health and Social Behavior, 28,* 306-319.

Wallace, J. (1996). Theory of 12-step-oriented treatment. In F. Rotgers, D.S. Keller & J. Morgenstein (Eds.), *Treating substance abuse: Theory and technique* (pp. 13-36). New York: Guilford.

Werner, P.D. (1993). A Q-sort measure of beliefs about abortion. *Educational and Psychological Measurement, 53,* 513-521.

AUTHORS' NOTES

Chau-kiu Cheung, PhD, is an assistant professor in the Department of Applied Social Studies, City University of Hong Kong. He is now undertaking research on moral values, school performance, service effectiveness, lay theorizing, caregiving, social networking, and the quality of life of various target populations in Hong Kong. His other publications appear in various journals of social psychology and sociology.

Tak-yan Lee, PhD, is an associate professor and fieldwork coordinator, Department of Applied Social Studies, City University of Hong Kong. His areas of research interest include civic education, adolescent and family, field instruction, youth work, and mass culture. He had more than eight years of experience working with children and youth and their families before taking up a teaching post.

Chak-man Lee, BSW, is a front-line social worker who has more than eight years of experience working with young people having problems with drugs, gangs, and low academic achievement.

The authors wish to thank Vic George for his valuable reorganization of the manuscript.

Address correspondence to Chau-kiu Cheung, Department of Applied Social Studies, City University of Hong Kong, Tat Chee Avenue, Kowloon, Hong Kong (E-mail: ssjacky@cityu.edu.hk).

Treating Substance Abusers in Correctional Contexts: New Understandings, New Modalities. Pp. 201-219.
© 2003 by The Haworth Press, Inc. All rights reserved.
10.1300/J076v37n03_11

A Crack Kid Grows Up:
A Clinical Case Report

SHERRI McCARTHY

Northern Arizona University-Yuma

THOMAS FRANKLIN WATERS

Northern Arizona University-Yuma

ABSTRACT During the early 1980s, use of crack cocaine by expectant mothers introduced U.S. schools and social agencies to a large cohort of children with attachment problems, attention and learning difficulties, hyperactivity and other abnormal behaviors. Research focused on the early characteristics and needs of so-called "crack kids," but little information about how these children are faring as they enter adulthood has been published. This paper presents a detailed four-year case study, including psychological profile, parent reports, school records, information from probation agencies and daily observations of an adolescent exposed to crack cocaine in utero. Information about social, emotional and intellectual development of the subject during late adolescence is the focus of this paper. Suggestions for preparing society to better deal with increasing numbers of young adults with similar profiles are also included. *[Article copies available for a fee from The Haworth Document Delivery Service: 1-800-HAWORTH. E-mail address: <docdelivery@haworthpress.com> Website: <http://www.HaworthPress. com> © 2003 by The Haworth Press, Inc. All rights reserved.]*

KEYWORDS Crack cocaine, case study, adolescent development, rehabilitation

"Crack baby" is a term commonly utilized in the U.S. to describe infants born to mothers who ingested rock cocaine while pregnant. Early research, often exaggerated or misrepresented by the popular media, heightened social concern to epidemic proportions resulting in a moral crusade to "save" infants from the addicted caregivers. A public fervor to prosecute and jail mothers who abused drugs during pregnancy developed, along with a despair that public education would be destroyed when these babies entered school. Biogenics, class politics and stereotypes of the "evil mother" shadowed the debates. The fervor has now faded, replaced by more thoughtful but often contradictory or confounded research on the developmental effects of in utero exposure to cocaine.

In 1987, it was estimated that as many as 375,000 infants born in the U.S. each year had been exposed to crack cocaine by maternal use (Besharov, 1990). Although many consider this estimate high (Gomby & Shiono, 1991), and there are probably no reliable national estimates of prenatal cocaine exposure (Frank, 1992), there are doubtless many adolescents and young adults today who were exposed to rock cocaine during gestation. Little information is available on how these maturing "crack kids" fare as they enter the passage to adulthood. It is our purpose to offer some insight into this passage by: (1) reviewing the existing literature on cocaine-exposed infants; (2) drawing implications from this research for maturing "crack kids"; and (3) providing data gathered during an intensive observational case study completed on one subject, a crack-exposed infant born in 1979, from the ages of 17 to 21 years. Following this, we will offer suggestions for rehabilitating "crack kids" who end up in the criminal justice system.

BACKGROUND RESEARCH

Physical Effects

Women who abuse cocaine during pregnancy may experience a variety of complications, including spontaneous abortions, stillbirths, ruptured placentas and premature delivery (Inciardi, Surratt & Saum, 1997). Because cocaine crosses the blood/brain barrier after passing through the placenta during pregnancy, it also potentially effects the developing fetal brain as well as other organs and tissues (Mayes, 1992). Since the fetal liver is not fully developed and cannot quickly eliminate the drug, it also has a far longer half-life in a fetus than in an adult (Chasnoff, 1987; Ewing, 1992). Documented consequences of exposure include impaired fetal growth, low birth weight and small head circumference. Respiratory and urinary tract difficulties also appear more common among cocaine-exposed infants (Chasnoff, 1986; 1988). Some studies also report birth defects of the kidneys, arms and heart (Cherukuri, 1988); however, these studies may not have accounted for synergistic effects of other teratogens used during pregnancy, such as alcohol. Cocaine also appears to be linked to the likelihood of Sudden Infant Death Syndrome (SIDS) (Chasnoff, 1986; Porat, Brodsky, Gianette & Hurt, 1994), although this relationship is uncertain due to the difficulty of separating out the multiple effects of poverty, cigarette smoking, alcohol use, poor nutrition and inadequate prenatal care from cocaine use (Zuckerman & Frank, 1992). Thus, studies do not agree regarding the increase of incidence of SIDS and other health problems among cocaine-exposed infants (Barton, Harrigan & Tse, 1995; Bauchner, 1988; Fulroth, Duran, Nicjerson & Espinoza, 1989) and are often difficult to interpret due to other risks present such as use of other teratogens and poor prenatal care. Regardless, there appears to be sufficient evidence to assume that "crack babies" are likely to be less healthy than other infants. Some researchers have claimed that difficulties seem to disappear as early as three years of age (Griffith, 1994) and others have noted that nutrition and environment after birth may account for either continued poor health or improvement. However, if crack exposure during infancy does have long-term effects on physical health, "crack kids" may be less healthy, overall, than their non-exposed peers during adolescence and early adulthood and may require more frequent medical care.

Socioemotional Effects

Because cocaine is a powerful central nervous system stimulant with lasting neurobehavioral effects, it can potentially retard social and emotional development. Mayes (1992) notes that potential manifestations include excessive crying, heightened reactivity to light and touch, delays in language development and lower intelligence. It has been difficult to demonstrate long-term behavioral, cognitive and language problems in children who were exposed prenatally to cocaine (Mentis & Lundgren, 1995). Because prenatal cocaine exposure was not widely recognized or researched until the mid-1980s, the study of neurological impairment related to use has a brief history and continued study is necessary to confirm or refute general clinical impressions (Inciardi, Surrett & Saum, 1997). Documented clinical impressions of crack-exposed infants include sleep dysfunction, irregularities in response to stimuli, excessive crying and fussiness (Dipietro, 1995). Most studies suggest these infants are more easily aroused but others have found cocaine-exposed infants to be more difficult to stimulate. Lester (1991) suggests this can be accounted for by the fact that the easily aroused infants are experiencing the effects of recent maternal cocaine use while the others are displaying the effect of chronic use on infant growth and development.

Studies employing tools such as the Brazelton Neonatal Behavioral Assessment Scale (NBAS) or the Bayley Scales of Infant Development (BSID) have mixed results. Dow-Edwards (1992) found that newborns exposed to crack had decreased interactive skills, short attention spans, comparatively depressed performance in psychomotor development and oversensitivity to stimulation, coping with stimulus by either frantic wails or sleep. Bateman (1993) reported brief tremors for the first 24 hours after birth. Mayes, Bornstein, Chawarska and Granger (1995) found evidence that visual information processing demonstrated increased arousal to stimuli which may exceed optimal levels for sustaining attention or processing information. Chasnoff, Griffith, Macgregor, Dirkes and Burns (1985) found that cocaine-exposed infants demonstrated poorer state regulation, orientation and motor performance than controls and presented more abnormal reflexes. Richardson, Hamel, Goldschmidt and Day (1996), in a carefully controlled study, found maternal cocaine use was significantly related to poorer autonomic stability, poorer motor maturity and tone and increased abnormal reflexes 2 days after birth. They suggest that infants exposed to cocaine may be more vulnerable to the stress of birth and exhibit a delayed recovery from that stress. Mentis and Lundgren (1995) suggest that explicit conclusions are difficult to reach from this data because measures used may not be sufficiently sensitive to identify other potential problems which may not manifest until later stages of development.

In a study of toddlers who had been exposed to crack cocaine while in utero, Howard, Beckwith, Rodning and Kropenske (1989) found that, compared to controls, subjects were emotionally and socially underdeveloped and had difficulty learning. Drug-exposed children did not show strong feelings of pleasure, anger or distress and appeared to be less purposeful and organized when playing. They also appeared unattached to their primary caregivers. During infancy, development of empathy is fostered by the affective relationship that develops between infant and caregiver (Barnett, 1987). Later, empathy develops when caregivers provide opportunities for children to experience a variety of emotions and encourage them to attend to the emotional experiences of others (Goldstein & Michaels, 1985). Lack of attachment combined with poor attention span may make it difficult for "crack kids" to develop empathy. Similarly, avoidant or ambivalent attachment appears to foster an external locus of control (Ainsworth, 1982; Guyot & Strehlow, 2000). Individuals with highly external loci of control assume that they have no control over their own actions or circumstances. From the perspective of these individuals, fate or destiny, those in power or other criteria determine the outcome of events. They do not see their own behavior or effort as having any effect on the events in their lives.

Implications of this research for later development of "crack kids" suggests lack of empathy and a highly external locus of control as defined by Rotter (1966) may be common characteristics as they mature. The current profile for Attention Deficit Hyperactivity Disorder (ADHD), a condition which has been increasingly common in recent years, also sounds strikingly consistent with this early research on "crack babies." Leichtman (1989) notes that parent/child attachment, internal representation of the world, empathy, self-soothing, self-regulation, self-esteem, values and competencies, learning and organizational strategies, social skills, responsibility and problem-solving are all difficulties encountered in a child with ADHD personality development. Martinez and Bournival (1995) note that ADHD children exhibit low cortical arousal as infants. Rapoport and Castellanos (1996) found evidence that ADHD children had significantly smaller right frontal brain regions and right striatum than controls. These findings seem consistent with the physiological and neurological data gathered on crack-exposed newborns and suggest that ADD or ADHD may be yet another manifestation of in utero crack exposure as children mature. This is not to suggest that ADD or ADHD is indicative of maternal cocaine use, as a variety of other factors may also contribute to the condition. However, one precursor to the condition may, indeed, be exposure to teratogens in utero, making it far more likely that "crack kids" will suffer from this condition than others.

Cognitive Effects

An ADD or ADHD profile markedly effects learning, cognition and educational success. Other cognitive developmental influences of cocaine exposure include delays in the acquisition of language skills, literacy and memory. In a study of 35 crack-exposed infants and 35 matched controls, van Baar and Graaff (1994) concluded that drug-exposed children tended to score lower on all general intelligence and language measures than controls and were functioning at a lower cognitive level as preschoolers. Similar studies by Mentis and Lundgren (1995) and Nulman (1994) provided similar results. However, cognitive assessments using general cognitive, verbal performance, quantitative and memory scales given by Hawley, Halle, Drasin and Thomas (1995) did not reveal significant differences between drug-exposed and non-drug-exposed children. Barone (1994) studied 26 cocaine-exposed children from 1 to 7 years of age who were placed in stable foster homes. She reported there were some noticeable delays but, overall, literacy patterns were developing in a manner similar to non-exposed children. It appears adverse cognitive effects may be mediated to some degree by a stable home environment and exacerbated by an unstable environment. Mayes (1992) suggested that a number of neurobehavioral differences between crack-exposed and non-exposed infants may disappear by 6 months of age, noting that the plasticity of the brain, combined with adequate caretaking, may compensate for some or all of the neurological insult. Zuckerman (1993) concurs. However, it seems to be evident that prenatal cocaine exposure does effect neurological functioning and is manifested by inappropriate response to stimulus, attentional impairments, language difficulties and learning problems. Such data suggests that difficulty in school, difficulty holding jobs and relatively low verbal intelligence scores may be characteristic of "crack kids" during adolescence and early adulthood.

Summary

No comparative studies of adolescents and young adults who were exposed to crack cocaine in utero are presently available. Based on the data gathered on cocaine-exposed infants and children, however, several likely characteristics can be extrapolated (see Table 1). Adolescents and young adults exhibiting several of these characteristics may have difficulty completing their schooling, holding jobs and functioning in society. Homelessness and incarceration may be likely potential outcomes for many members of this cohort unless intensive early intervention is continued throughout adolescence and early adulthood. Given the characteristics likely to present themselves during adolescence and early adulthood such as a strong desire to "fit in" with peers, low impulse control, low self-esteem and poor self-monitoring ability, prison is a likely future outcome for this group, but not necessarily a useful one. The case study presented here supports this conclusion.

☐ ***Table 1: Characteristics of Individuals Exposed to Cocaine in Utero Based on Previous Research***

Developmental Delays (Cognitive and Socioemotional)
Relatively Low Verbal Ability
Attention and/or Memory Deficits
Hyperactivity
Learning Difficulties
Generally Disorganized
Poor Motor Coordination
Some Antisocial Tendencies
Heightened Reactivity to Light and Touch
Sleep Dysfunction
Respiratory and Urinary Difficulties
Moodiness
Seizures
Inability to Bond with Peers or Parents
Inconsolability
Less Social Interactivity
Growth Retardation
Low Impulse Control
Poor Self-Monitoring Ability
Inappropriate Response to Stimuli
Oversensitivity to Stimuli
Behavior Consistent with ADHD Profile
Strong Desire to "Fit In" Socially
Very Literal Interpretations of Information
Low Self-Esteem
Low Affect/Low Arousal Level

METHODOLOGY

Subject

The subject of this case study is a young American male of Scottish and German heritage. He was born in January 1979, in southern California. His father was a college-educated U.S. Naval officer; his mother had also attended college but, according to interview data gathered from the subject, the subject's father and his maternal grandmother, his mother was addicted to crack cocaine and smoked it regularly throughout her pregnancy. Despite this, the subject was delivered normally, only two weeks prior to full term. He was healthy and weighed approximately 6.5 lbs. at birth. He is currently 6'3" tall, slim and muscular.

At the age of 2, he reportedly ingested a rock of crack cocaine from his mother's "stash" and was hospitalized for several days. His parents subsequently divorced, ostensibly because of his mother's addiction. His father remarried and acquired custody when the subject was 4 years of age. The subject attended elementary school at a Department of Defense school in Japan, where his father was stationed. He was retained in second grade. He next attended middle school in the Washington, D.C., area, where he was diagnosed as ADHD. He moved to a small city in the southwestern U.S. in early adolescence where he remained until being sent to prison at the age of 21.

The subject was unable to finish high school, but obtained a G.E.D. at the age of 20. He reports being close to his stepmother who "tried hard to be a Mom but had problems of her own." He has two half-brothers, over ten years younger than he is. He reports that he enjoys spending time with them and says he "loves my brothers really a lot–kids are so cool!" He viewed his childhood as normal, although he reports his father was "very strict, had a lot of rules and got mad at me a lot." He reports still admiring and loving his father and reports that "I understand why he doesn't like me. I wish I hadn't disappointed him so much but I guess I just can't help it." The subject has had no contact with his birth mother (now dead) for the last eighteen years. His stepmother died of a heroin overdose when he was 17 years of age. His father kicked him out of the house on his eighteenth birthday, telling him it was "time he became a man." He was homeless and lived on the street for approximately one month before being invited to participate in this study. He and his father had no contact for approximately one year after that time. They now have a limited but civil relationship. He reported to his probation officer on one occasion that "I think I need a lot of counseling because of all that stuff, but as long as I have my friends, I'll be okay."

The subject reported his long-range goals at the time the study began as "I want to get a job I like, maybe doing something with science where I can take things apart and mix chemicals or in a hospital . . . and to marry and have a family."

Instrumentation

A variety of data points were used and triangulated. Extensive interviews with the subject, several of his friends and peers, his father and his grandmother were conducted. His teachers, counselors, employers and probation officers were also interviewed. These interviews were conducted over a three-year period and combined with extensive notes based on systematic observations. High school records, standardized test scores, police records, letters written to friends, personal journals and probation records were also available. In addition, the subject completed a variety of tests for purposes of this study, including the Wechsler Adult Intelligence Scales-III (WAIS-III), WAIS-Short Form, Myers-Briggs Personality Type Indicator (MBTI), Rotter Incomplete Sentence Blank, IAR Scales, Importance of Goals Scale, Adolescent Health Survey and HSPQ. Trained graduate students who were unaware of the purpose of the study or of the subject's background administered these tests.

Procedure

This is a report of a case study based on clinical observation in the tradition of Piaget and other psychologists. One of the authors encountered the subject through his interactions with teenage children, 3 to 5 years his junior, in 1996. Upon becoming aware of his homelessness and his desire to finish high school, he was invited into the author's home. At that time, he was 18 years of age although developmentally he exhibited characteristics of a child in early adolescence rather than a young adult. Shortly thereafter, as the author became aware of his history and profile, he was asked if he would be willing to be a subject in a case study, provided his confidentiality was assured. He agreed willingly, noting "that sounds fun; I've always liked science and maybe it will help somebody." Observational notes covering 1996-97 were completed retrospectively. From March 1997 until January 2000, clinical notes were kept on a daily basis. These included observations of activities, conversations, responses to events, diet, health, sleep patterns, substance use, peer interaction and any other information that seemed relevant. Data was also provided to the researchers by the subject's probation officers, counselors and teachers, and information from interviews with his family members was included. Many of the observations gathered on this subject during late adolescence and early adulthood seem to mirror the findings of research on crack-exposed infants as they may be expected to manifest at a later developmental stage, remarkably well.

RESULTS

A brief narrative summary of the data collected as described above related to physical, social, emotional and cognitive development appears below. Tables 2-4 summarize major relevant observed characteristics in light of characteristics expected from research on crack-exposed infants and children.

☐ *Table 2: Characteristics of Infants Exposed to Cocaine in Utero Based on Previous Research Which Are Evident in the Subject During Early Adulthood*

Developmental Delays (Cognitive and Socioemotional)
Relatively Low Verbal Ability
Attention Deficits with Hyperactivity
Learning Difficulties
Generally Disorganized
Poor Motor Coordination
Some Antisocial Tendencies
Heightened Reactivity to Light
Heightened Reactivity to Touch
Sleep Dysfunction
Respiratory and Urinary Difficulties

☐ *Table 3: Characteristics of Infants Exposed to Cocaine in Utero Based on Previous Research Which Are Absent in the Subject During Early Adulthood*

Seizures
Inability to Bond with Peers
Inconsolability
Low Social Interactivity
Growth Retardation

☐ *Table 4: Characteristics of the Subject Which May Have Been Influenced by Exposure to Cocaine*

Divergent/Creative Thought Patterns (Inappropriate Response to Stimuli)
Musical Ability (Heightened Sensitivity to Sound/Oversensitivity to Stimuli)
High Need for Structure (Consistent with ADHD Profile)
Strong Desire to "Fit in" Socially
Very Literal Interpretations of Information (Suggesting Developmental Delay)
Good Sense of Humor (Inappropriate Response to Stimuli)
Pleasant and Sunny Disposition (Low Affect/Low Arousal Level)
Perception of Self as "Bad" or "Evil" (Low Self-Esteem)
Abuse of Marijuana, Hallucinogens, Alcohol and Tobacco (Attempt to Self-Medicate)
Avoidance of and Opposition to Use of All Other Illicit Drugs (Oversensitivity to Stimuli)
Strong Desire to "Stand Out" or "Be Unique" in Some Way (Developmental Delay)
Pro-Social Interactions with Peers, Friends, Family and Pets
Antagonistic Towards Law Enforcement Officials (Consistent with ADHD/OD Profile)
Strong Desire for Successful Education, Marriage and Family
Strong Desire to Work and to Contribute to Society
Difficulty Holding a Job (Cognitive, Motor & Socioemotional Developmental Delays)
Difficulty in School (Cognitive Delay/ADHD Profile)

Physical Effects

As noted earlier, it may be expected that early physical and neurological stress imposed by cocaine exposure can impair health. The subject's diagnosis as ADHD may well be related to early exposure. In addition, compared to other young adults with similar lifestyles, he appeared far more prone to colds, pneumonia, accidents and infections, and made frequent visits to medical facilities for these conditions. Early evidence of respiratory and urinary difficulty and of poor motor coordination appears, in this case, to be long lasting. He reported, on several occasions "I get sick a lot," and "I have a lot of accidents and I'd like to play sports but I've never been very good at running or catching things."

The subject appears to have a rapid metabolism. He consumes large quantities of food, yet remains lean and reports being constantly hungry. His preferences are for healthy food. Fruits, vegetables, juices and pasta were preferred menu choices. He sleeps comparatively little, having difficulty sleeping at night and generally remaining awake until 2 or 3 a.m. He was generally awake by 7 a.m. each morning during the years observed and occasionally took short afternoon naps. Sleep dysfunction, apparently, also was a lasting effect of inutero exposure in this case. It should be noted, however, that the subject did not view his health or his sleep patterns as problematic or different from others.

Socioemotional Effects

The subject exhibited delays in social development. He gravitated toward peers who were much younger, chronologically. In fact, he often reported viewing the first author's son, nearly four years his junior, as "like a big brother to me." That son also noted that the subject "sure seems a lot younger than me." The subject seemed to relate best to friends between the ages of 11 and 14 (early adolescence) even at the age of 21. His preferred pastimes included music, video games, activities with large, mixed-sex peer groups, disassembling mechanical objects, creating strange chemical compounds to "kill bugs," and riding a bicycle. These behavior patterns are characteristic of early, not late, adolescence.

Observations indicated the subject was frequently preoccupied with justice and fairness and had a very literal view of the world and of good and evil. He perceived himself as evil. He demonstrated tremendous concern for and loyalty to friends and family and especially enjoyed participating in family meals and outings. He reported "macaroni and cheese with tomatoes is my favorite food because that's what my (step)mom used to make when things were going good and she was trying to be a mom." He also loved caring for and spending time with his younger brothers and considered his peer group "my best family." He often demonstrated sensitivity to others. He saw himself as a peace-loving flower child who "would only fight if I absolutely had to, because I think it is wrong." He did, however, report that he had, on occasion, needed to fight to establish himself in new neighborhoods or to "stand up for myself against gangs and stuff" and according to peer accounts, motor coordination aside, he was a good "street-fighter" who was "safe to be around 'cuz gang kids leave us alone if he's there." He liked "taking care of his friends and of people that are good to me." He reported that "playing music is the best thing in the world for me. It really helps me cope and calms me down." He always appeared relatively calm, demonstrating either good emotional control or relatively flat effect. He displayed a ready smile, good sense of humor, interesting perspective on many issues and generally sunny disposition.

He often noted that "I really want to get married and have a family and take good care of them." During the course of the study, he had only one serious romantic relationship. It lasted for approximately six months before the girl, four years younger than he and equally troubled, albeit for different reasons, broke it off. He reported "I'll still always love her and take care of her." She later became a teen, unwed mother (the father was a friend of the subject's, now also in prison). The subject remained helpful and supportive, often caring for her child, trying to "cheer her up" and in other ways supporting her. He still writes to her frequently from prison. Although she has yet to return a letter, he states "she's the only one for me." He is almost chivalrous in his general treatment of women.

The subject demonstrates strong contradictory urges "to fit in and earn respect" and to "stand out and be really unique." This is not inconsistent with early adolescent development. In his peer group, he is more a follower than a leader in activities even though he associates with younger peers.

He admittedly "is really a stoner and need my pot." He also frequently used hallucinogens and drank alcohol. He is adamantly opposed to any other illegal drug use, however. "I've seen what that stuff does to people–no way! If one of my friends was doing meth or smoking crack, I'd take it away and flush it or even turn them in."

Based on the data collected, he did not seem to demonstrate major problems with attachment. He attributed many events to "luck" or "karma," demonstrating a more external locus of control, but often accepted responsibility for his actions. He did not seem particularly aggressive, violent, antisocial or insensitive, although cruelty to animals was observed on more than one occasion. Other destructive tendencies noted were a penchant for "killing bugs" and a habit of disassembling mechanical objects.

Cognitive Effects

Disorganization was apparent. Care for personal property was chaotic; the subject consistently forgot even such simple tasks as closing doors and turning out lights, although he responded well to a structured behavior-management program using social praise and token reinforcement. He seemed to respond well to highly structured situations and short, specific orders but had difficulty with complex directions. Although friendly, he was not highly verbal and, although he had a unique way of expressing his feelings, he often had difficulty doing so. He had been retained in elementary school and was a "fifth-year senior" in high school when he was first displaced from his home. Due to several events (described in Outcomes, below) he was unable to finish high school, although he was very motivated to do so. His teachers reported that "he tries really hard," "he likes and needs a lot of attention," and "he can learn; in fact he's pretty good at science compared to some kids, but he has a hard time studying and doing homework."

He was persistent with his studies, and seemed almost oblivious to his difficulties. "Oh, don't worry, I can help you with your homework," he eagerly told a friend who was complaining about his Freshman Algebra class on one occasion. "I've already taken that class 3 times, so I know the stuff really good by now!" Standardized testing done during his senior year of high school indicated he was reading at approximately a ninth-grade level and his math skills were at approximately the eighth-grade level. He scored at approximately the 25th percentile, overall, compared to his chronological peers. He was eventually able to pass the exam for a General Education Diploma (G.E.D.) after approximately six months of tutoring and preparation.

Vocational and Life Skills Implications

The subject had difficulty functioning in the workplace. He maintained a job at a fast-food restaurant for approximately one month. He was fired, according to his supervisor, "because of constant illness and because he seemed to get flustered when things got busy. During rush hours, he couldn't count change correctly if he was at the cash register and he couldn't produce food quickly enough when he was in the kitchen. He did okay during training or when things were slow. He was a nice kid and he tried really hard, but it just didn't work out." He next worked as a taxi driver but, after two accidents in his first week of work, was again dismissed. He worked on construction sights, first mixing concrete. "He was so clumsy," reported his supervisor. "He tripped over things and spilled things all the time. He was a hazard on the worksite and probably cost us $1000.00 in broken equipment and wasted supplies." He also apprenticed briefly as a drywall finisher. "I could train him if I had enough time," reported his supervisor. "He had a good eye and he had the height, strength and speed necessary. He needed a lot of direction, though." The job he held the longest was in a warehouse, loading crates of fertilizer and other chemicals for delivery. He eventually quit because "being around all that stuff all the time was making me sick. My skin stung and I couldn't breathe." Currently, in prison, he is employed cleaning bathrooms. "I think I'm pretty good at it, but it doesn't pay very well," he reported in a letter to a friend.

He was always willing to help with household tasks, especially when structured chore lists and operant behavior management strategies were used. He was best at simple tasks, however, and needed constant direction and step-by-step instructions to complete assigned chores. His attention deficits were noticeable; even when playing music, which he loved, it was rare for him to be able to finish a song without stopping in the middle. His memory for events, however, seemed good. He often demonstrated novel, creative problem-solving skills, especially in social situations and enjoyed disassembling various household items and reassembling the parts together into "new machines."

Psychometric Observations

On tests of intelligence (WAIS-Short Form and WAIS-III) scores were in the normal range, with full scale IQ of 102 and 106, respectively. A significant discrepancy in verbal and performance scores was evident however; verbal scores were over one standard deviation below average, while performance scores were over one standard deviation above. The IAR Scale (Rotter, 1966) indicated a moderately high external locus of control. The Adolescent Health Questionnaire and the Rotter Incomplete Sentences Blank both resulted in normal profiles consistent with age. The Meyers Briggs Type Indicator resulted in a profile of ESFP–extroverted, sensory-oriented, feeling rather than rational and non-judgmental. The High School Personality Questionnaire results were midrange (sten of 4 to 6) on all factors except A (sten 3–reserved and detached); B (sten 3–concrete rather than abstract thinking); D (sten 7–impatient and easily distracted); I (sten 7–sensitive and intuitive); O (sten 7–self-blaming and guilt-prone), and Q2 (sten 1–a "joiner" and follower who is easily influenced by others). The Importance of Goals Scales revealed that Interpersonal Goals were most important to the subject, followed by career and reputation.

The psychometric profiles are, on surface observation, quite normal. Closer examination, especially of WAIS score discrepancies and the High School Personality Questionnaire personality factors are, however, consistent with early research on "crack kids," demonstrating relatively low verbal ability, distractibility and low self-esteem.

Present Outcomes

When the subject was 16, he was involved in a break-in. According to his own report and the report of several peers, his involvement was not intentional. "It was one of those times when his Dad had kicked him out of the house because he forgot to feed the dog or something," reported one source. "It was kinda late and he was tired and didn't have anywhere to go and he ran into this kid who said 'Hey, come with me, I have a place.' He was supposedly watching these people's trailer for them or something. He went and there was a big party going on. He pretty much just slept on the couch. But they really trashed the place while he was asleep and the cops came and when they got there it was just him and a couple of little kids that they caught inside 'cuz everybody else ran out the back. He got blamed for it 'cuz he was the oldest and the whole thing was on film, too. His Dad said to the cops he probably did it 'cuz he was no good."

The subject was not charged with the crime until after his eighteenth birthday. Despite the fact that it had occurred nearly two years earlier, he was tried as an adult. He was arrested and locked up until his trial less than a month from his projected high school graduation date. His absences from school made it impossible for him to finish his educational goal. Undaunted, he reported "jail wasn't that bad," and began studying for his G.E.D. As a result of his trial, he was sentenced to intensive probation and required to pay over $60,000.00 in restitution over the course of his life. After serving over two-and-one-half years on probation successfully, he was issued a violation by a newly assigned probation officer when a urine screen tested positive for marijuana use. He was sentenced to 5 years in prison, where he currently resides. His initial response was characteristically sunny and concrete–"You know what they say; if you're gonna do the crime than you gotta do the time." He advises his friends in letters from jail to "stay out of trouble; you don't want to go the route I've gone. Stupidity is why I'm here. I rebelled against the system and look where I'm at. I have learned from my mistakes." His letters have remained generally upbeat; he has access to a guitar and has formed a band with other inmates. He reports that they may have a CD made soon. He reads frequently, is happy that he has a job cleaning toilets and is "making lots of new friends."

Other indicators in letters, however, suggest that these "new friends," combined with his high influenceability and the desire to fit in documented elsewhere, may be part of a process that obliterates any chance for a normal, prosocial life for this young man when he is released. He is learning how to make "homemade acid" and getting tattoos. He is learning "I have to fight to stand up for myself." His formerly sunny disposition is being replaced by bouts with depression. "I feel so alone, confined to my own hell," he writes in a letter to a friend. "I'm left to rot in my own depressions and hatreds of life, locked in a closet. I sit here and do the same shit everyday. My young life has grown old. I wish I could take a step forward into the good side. Sometimes I want to die and be free from my terrors and fears, but one thing keeps me here alive and that is the thought of being able to be with you and all the others I care about that also care for me again some day."

DISCUSSION

Implications for Educators

The prosocial tendencies, motivation to succeed and good memory this subject demonstrates suggest that educators who are in fear of "crack kids in the classroom" may be functioning to create self-fulfilling prophecies rather than legitimately responding to student needs, as some researchers have suggested (Best, 1994). Although special techniques may be required, these students can certainly be taught.

Providing a structured learning environment, breaking down assignments into small steps, utilizing task analysis to sequence learning and providing consistent reinforcement in the forms of praise and positive social recognition all appear to be promising strategies. Encouraging positive peer interaction through cooperative group work also may be beneficial. Utilizing school counselors, school psychologists and other community resources to provide additional life skills training, utilizing a cognitive-behavioral model, is also recommended.

Social Implications

There may be a strong underlying relationship between the current plethora of ADD- and ADHD-diagnosed students in American public schools and maternal drug use that bears further investigation. It is worth noting that the subject described here was not in any way reminiscent of the "crack kids" portrayed in the media. He was not Black or Hispanic. He was not born to a single, uneducated mother in the inner city and was not raised in poverty. Overall, despite obvious deficits, he experienced good parenting in a stable, structured home throughout most of his childhood. He had adequate nutrition, good medical care and education.

This case supports the hypothesis that much of the early "crack data" was politically motivated, reflecting racial bias, gender bias and classism. There are undoubtedly many other cases like this young man–crack kids born to white, middle and upper class homes who were missed in all of the early hype when data was collected primarily in treatment centers and public health facilities. A large cohort of "hidden" cases may exist, suggesting estimates should be higher, rather than lower, for incidence of maternal drug use.

It is also worth noting that many characteristics noted in "crack babies" seemed to have lasting effects on this subject. Developmental delays, poor health and coordination and cognitive deficits seemed lasting. On the other hand, the more labile emotional traits such as failure to attach, inability to bond, aggressiveness and lack of control were lacking. Perhaps this suggests that a nurturing environment more easily ameliorates social outcomes than physical and cognitive outcomes. As Zuckerman and Frank (1994) note, intervention focused on parenting is well worth pursuing and very effective.

Lasting physical and cognitive outcomes may be problematic for the social welfare system, especially as homelessness may be a particular problem for this group. Additional vocational counseling and jobs skills training may be needed to help this generation of "crack babies" as they enter adulthood. These services should perhaps also be coordinated with criminal justice organizations, where many of this group may find themselves.

Implications for U.S. Criminal Justice System

An arbitrary, punitive criminal justice system may have, in this case, irrevocably damaged the chances of recovery of this young man who, otherwise, seemed to be doing fairly well in his delayed development toward a normal life. The behavioral tendencies predicted by in utero exposure to crack cocaine are probably more likely to lead to arrest of "crack kids" than of non-exposed adolescents and adults. We speculate that many of the current prison population in the U.S. under the age of 25 may, indeed be "crack kids grown up." If this is indeed the case, it would behoove society to find better ways of dealing with these individuals than incarceration. Cognitive-behavioral training programs, peer mentoring, appropriate social support and education programs that lead to productive, albeit somewhat delayed, self-supporting lives would seem to be a wiser approach than supporting this group at taxpayer expense in a system that is likely to exacerbate rather than ameliorate problem behaviors when the focus is not on rehabilitation.

Additional research comparing crack-exposed and non-crack-exposed adolescents, though fraught with methodological problems and difficult to conduct, is warranted given the lasting nature and extensive impact of this problem. Additionally, research on young prison populations and incarcerated juveniles is an avenue worth pursuing. The characteristics noted in this case study make adolescents and young adults who were exposed in utero to crack cocaine, methamphetamine and/or excessive alcohol particularly at risk for homelessness, criminal behavior and a lack of community support. This may result in incarceration for a substantial percentage of this group. A large-scale retrospective study of prison populations is warranted, and it may be important for psychologists who are evaluating probationers, parolees and inmates to gather information on previous exposure to substances in utero and on behavioral risks associated with such exposure in order to better tailor treatment plans to the particular needs of "crack kids grown up." Focusing on strengths rather than weaknesses or deficits and providing highly structured environments with necessary training and support services seems warranted.

REFERENCES

Baar, A.V. & Graaf, F. (1994). Cognitive development of preschool age infants of drug-dependent mothers. *Developmental Medical Child Neurology, 36, 12,* 1036-75.
Barnett, M.A. (1987). Empathy and related responses in children. In N. Eisenberg & J. Strayer (Eds.), *Empathy and its development,* 146-162.
Barone, D. (1994). Myths about crack babies. *Educational Leadership, 52, 2,* 67-8.

Barton, S.J., Harrington, N. & Tse, J. (1995). Prenatal cocaine exposure: Implications for practice, policy development and needs for future research. *Journal of Prenatal Nursing, 15, 1,* 10-22.

Bateman, D.A. (1993). *The effects of intrauterine cocaine exposure in newborns. American Journal of Public Health, 83, 2,* 190-193.

Bauchner, H. (1988). Cocaine use during pregnancy: prevalence and correlates. *Pediatrics, 82, 6,* 888-895.

Bender, S.L., Word, C.O., Diclemente, R.J., Crittendon, M.R., Persuad, N.A. & Ponton, L.E. (1995). The developmental implications of prenatal and/or postnatal crack cocaine exposure in preschool children: A preliminary report. *Developmental and Behavioral Pediatrics, 16, 6,* 418-424.

Best, J.B. (Ed.) (1994). *Troubling children: Studies of children and social problems.* New York: Aldine de Gruyter.

Chasnoff, I.J. (1986). Prenatal drug exposure: Effects on neonatal and infant growth and development. *Neurobehavioral Toxicology and Teratolology, 8, 4,* 357-362.

Chasnoff, I.J. (1989). Drug use and women: Establishing a standard of care. In *Prenatal abuse of licit and illicit drugs. Annals of the New York Academy of Sciences, 5, 62,* 208-210.

Chasnof, I., Griffith, D., Macgregor, S., Dirkes, L. & Burns, K. (1989). Temporal patterns of cocaine use in pregnancy: Perinatal outcomes. *Journal of the American Medical Association, 261,* 1741-44.

Dipietro, J. (1995). Reactivity and regulation in cocaine exposed neonates. *Infant Behavior and Development, 18, 4,* 407-414.

Dow-Edwards, D. (1992). *Perinatal substance abuse: Research findings and clinical implications.* Baltimore, MD: Johns Hopkins University Press.

Frank, D., Bresnahan, K. & Zuckerman, B. (1993). Maternal cocaine use: Impact on child health & development. *Advances in Pediatrics, 40, 1,* 65-99.

Fulroth, R., Duran, D., Nicjerson, A. & Espinoza, J. (1989). Perinatal outcome of infants exposed to cocaine and/or heroin in utero. *American Journal of Disabilities in Children, 143, 8,* 905-10.

Goldstein, A.P. & Michaels, G.Y. (1985). *Empathy: Development, training and consequences.* New Jersey: Erlbaum.

Griffith, D. (1994). Three year outcome of children exposed prenatally to drugs. *Journal of the Academy of Child and Adolescent Psychiatry, 33, 1,* 20-27.

Guyot, G., & Strehlow, A. (2000, April). *Parent attachment, adult attachment style and locus of control.* Paper presented at the 2000 Annual Meeting of the Southwestern Psychological Association, Dallas, TX.

Hawley, T., Halle, L., Drasin, A, & Thomas, S. (1995). Children of addicted mothers: Effects of the crack epidemic on the caregiving environment and the development of preschoolers. *American Journal of Orthopsychiatry, 65, 3,* 364-379.

Howard, J., Beckworth, L., Rodning, C. & Kropenske, V. (1989). The development of young children of substance-abusing parents: Insights from seven years of intervention and research. *Bulletin of the National Center for Clinical Infant Programs, 9, 5,* 8-12.

Inciardi, J.A., Surrett, H.L. & Saum, C.A. (1997). Cocaine-exposed infants: Social. Legal and public policy issues. *Drugs, Health and Public Policy Series, Volume 5.* London: Sage Publications.

Lester, B. (1991). Neurobehavioral syndromes in cocaine-exposed newborn infants. *Child Development, 62, 4,* 694-705.

Martinez, A. & Bournival, B. (1995). ADHD: The tip of the iceberg. *ADHD Report, 3, 6.*

Mayes, L. C. (1992). The problem of prenatal cocaine exposure: A rush to judgment. *Journal of the American Medical Association, 267, 3,* 406-408.

Mayes, L.C., Bornstein, B., Chaworska, C. & Granger, G. (1995). Information processing and developmental assessments in 3-month-old infants exposed prenatally to cocaine. *Pediatrics, 95, 4,* 539-545.

Mentis, M. & Lundgren, N. (1995). Effects of prenatal exposure to cocaine and associated risk factors on language development. *Journal of Speech and Hearing Research, 38, 6,* 1303-1318.

Nulman, I. (1994). Neurodevelopment of adopted children exposed in utero to cocaine. *Canadian Medical Association Journal, 151, 11,* 1591-1597.

Porat, R., Brodsky, D., Gianette, J. & Hurt, H. (1994). Prenatally exposed to cocaine: Does the label matter? *Journal of Early Intervention, 182, 2,* 119-130.

Rapoport, J. & Castellanos, J. (1995, Nov.). *Neurological profiles of children with ADD.* Paper presented at the C.H.A.D.D. Conference, Washington, D.C.

Richardson, G.A., Hamel, S. Goldschmidt, L. & Day, N. (1996). The effects of prenatal cocaine use on neonatal neurobehavioral status. *Neurotoxicology & Teretotology, 18, 5,* 519-528.

Rotter, J.B. (1966). Generalized expectation for internal versus external control of reinforcement. *Psychological Monographs, 80,* 609.

Zuckerman, B. (1993). Children exposed to cocaine prenatally: Pieces of the puzzle. *Neurotoxicology & Teratology, 15, 5,* 281-312.

Zuckerman, B. & Frank, D.A. (1992). Crack kids: Not broken. *Pediatrics, 82, 2,* 337-339.

Zuckerman, B. & Frank, D.A. (1994). Prenatal cocaine & marijuana exposure: Research and clinical implications. In I. Zaigon & T. Slotkin (Eds.), *Maternal Substance Abuse and Neurodevelopment.* New York: Academic Press.

AUTHORS' NOTES

Sherri McCarthy, PhD, is an associate professor of Educational Psychology at Northern Arizona University-Yuma. She holds a PhD in educational psychology with an emphasis in human development and cognition. She teaches courses in adolescent psychology, developing critical thinking skills, behavior management and personality adjustment. Her research focuses on teaching critical thinking and coping skills and on applications of psychology to education and criminal justice. She has written books on bereavement counseling and special education issues and recently had a chapter published on educational strategies to reduce the likelihood that adolescents will commit acts of terrorism in *The Psychology of Terrorism, Vol. 3* (Greenwood Press, 2002), edited by Chris Stout. Dr. McCarthy is active in APA's International Psychology Project through Division 2 and served on the organizing committee for the first international conference on the teaching of psychology for applied settings in St. Petersburg, Russia.

Thomas Franklin Waters, PhD, is an associate professor of Criminal Justice at Northern Arizona University-Yuma. He earned his PhD in criminal justice from the

University of Arizona with additional training from the University of Denver and the National Institute of Corrections. He has worked in rehabilitation programs in several prisons throughout the U.S. He recently completed a sabbatical project comparing opportunities for careers in criminal justice agencies for women in U.S. and Mexican agencies. Dr. Waters teaches courses in a variety of areas, including drug issues and the law, research methods in criminal justice and other current topics. He is active in the criminal justice community, cooperating with juvenile and adult probation agencies and police agencies throughout Arizona in a variety of projects and program evaluations.

Portions of this study were presented at the 53rd Conference of the International Council of Psychologists in Padua, Italy, and at the 2nd International Conference on Child and Adolescent Mental Health in Kuala Lumpur, Malaysia. The authors would like to thank the Yuma County Adult Probation Department for their continued partnership and support conducting research on applications of psychology to prisoner rehabilitation.

Address correspondence to Dr. Sherri McCarthy, Department of Educational Psychology, Counseling & Human Relations, Northern Arizona University-Yuma, PO Box 6236, Yuma, AZ 85366 (E-mail: sherri.mccarthy@nau.edu).

Index of Names and Topics